THE FOREVER GARDEN

Cara Rosehope has an honours degree in biochemistry, and a graduate diploma in horticulture from VCAH Burnley. She runs a Melbourne-based gardening consultancy specialising in adapting gardens for retirement. She is currently researching for a postgraduate degree on the spiritual value of gardening.

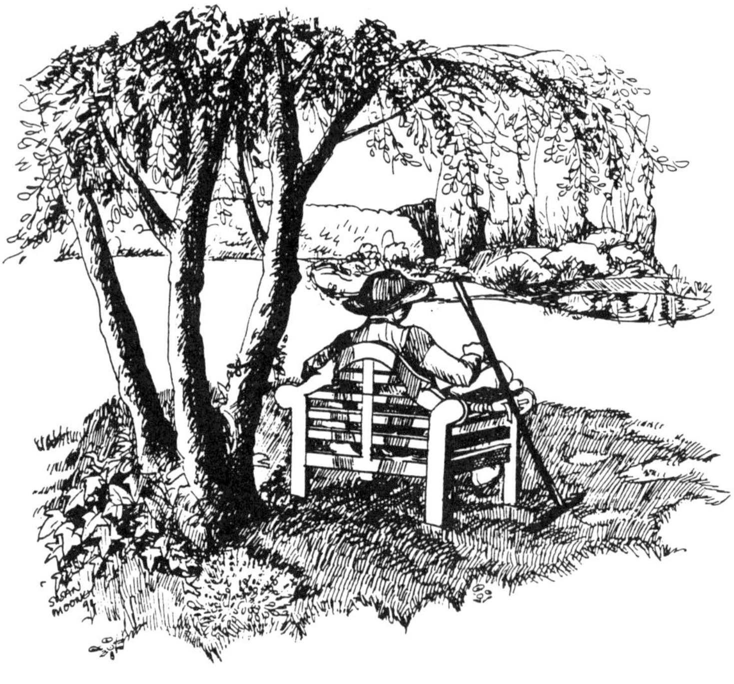

The Forever Garden

Creating an Easy-Care Garden

CARA ROSEHOPE

HYLAND HOUSE

First published in Australia in 1996 by
Hyland House Publishing Pty Limited
Hyland House
387-389 Clarendon Street
South Melbourne
Victoria 3205

National Library of Australia
Cataloguing-in-publication data:

Rosehope, Cara, 1949– .
The forever garden: creating an easy-care garden.

Bibliography.
Includes index.
ISBN 1 875657 70 3.

1. Gardens—Australia. 2. Low maintenance gardening—Australia. I. Title.

635.0994

Illustrated by Susan Mooney
Typeset in Australia by Solo Typesetting, South Australia
Printed in Hong Kong by Dai Nippon Printing Co. (HK) Ltd.

Contents

List of Illustrations

Acknowledgements

The seeds for this book were sown some years ago. Then I was doing maintenance gardening for people in their homes. Many of my clients were elderly and were no longer able to garden; some told me how much they missed it. The first time I heard this it went through me like a bolt of lightning and I realised just what a loss it would be to me if I could no longer garden. From that time on I began to hunt out ways of making gardening easier for the less able-bodied. Studying Horticultural Therapy as part of a Graduate Diploma in Horticulture put me in touch with a wealth of information about gardening within the Horticultural Therapy movement. It also made me aware that very little of this information ever came the way of the home gardener. This book is an attempt to put that to rights.

I was most fortunate in having one of my early newspaper articles come to the attention of Anne Godden from Hyland House, who then approached me to write the book that till then I had only dared dream of; I would like to thank Anne for her vision and for her enthusiasm for this project. I would like also to thank Nerissa Greenfield for making the editorial process a pleasure, Al Knight for his thoughtful design, and the others at Hyland House for their cheerful and friendly assistance.

I would like to convey my warmest gratitude to Susan Mooney, illustrator-extraordinare. Not only did she convert my vague descriptions and wild gesticulations into apt and charming drawings, but she did so with a good will and efficiency that was truly remarkable.

Thanks to friends and family who encouraged and supported me while I wrote the book, especially to John Holden for reading and editing my first drafts. Thanks also to my children, particularly Phoebe, who showed great forbearance during the writing process when much of her home life was placed 'on hold'.

I would like also to express my gratitude to the following people and organisations who contributed to this book: *Independent Living Centres* throughout Australia who responded to my requests for information about locally available tools and gardening aids; *Technical Aid for the Disabled— Victoria* for information on TAD country-wide; Sam Schirmer for her help with the pre-gardening exercises; the tool manufacturers and distributors who responded to my requests to 'road test' their tools.

Finally, I would like to thank all the older gardeners who have shared their love of gardening with me over the years, both those who are included in this book and those who are not; long may they garden.

Cara Rosehope
June 1996

In memory of Hope Elizabeth Pringle,
who missed her garden terribly.

1
Gardening as We Age

No occupation is as delightful to me as the culture of the earth, and no culture comparable to that of the garden. I am still devoted to the garden. But though an old man, I am but a young gardener.

THOMAS JEFFERSON

MORE AND MORE OF US ARE MARCHING ON TOWARDS RETIREMENT; IN developed countries world-wide the population is steadily greying. Today there are unprecedented numbers of retirees, and when the post-war Baby Boomers hit retirement age early in the twenty-first century there will be an abrupt leap in the number of people over the age of retirement. It is estimated that, by the year 2031, around one quarter of all Australians will be sixty years or older.

Already this growth in the number of retirees is bearing fruit. Third Agers have become the fastest growing market in the western world, and they now find themselves being wooed (and even occasionally catered for) by insurance companies, holiday tour firms, land developers and publishers alike. The field of geriatrics, too, has become of much greater interest to health workers, both professionally and, presumably, personally. While still not quite 'flavour of the month', gerontology has become at least respectable, and our knowledge of the ageing process has grown accordingly. A further consequence of the swelling number of superannuees is an increased awareness that retirement has much to offer. We can expect to spend as much as a third of our lives post-retirement, and thus there is a strong need to plan for, and take charge of, this stage of our lives.

For many of us as we grow older, gardening becomes of great importance; a good many of us will experience a veritable explosion of gardening activity upon retirement. Time can now be found for those things that we could never quite get round to before, be they bold new schemes or modest improvements. A number of us will move from the homes in which we raised our families; new gardening adventures will take place in smaller, more limited spaces.

Most of us will retire in possession of good health and a fair degree of strength. We will, however, be aware that we may need to make some changes, for most by then will have found it necessary to make some concessions to the passage of time. Advances in modern medicine mean that we are living longer while enjoying better health. Today we have a clearer understanding of the influence that life-style has on our well-being; there is much that we can do for ourselves towards preserving health and vigour.

Despite these advances, there is still some loss of abilities that occurs as we age. These commonly include a loss of strength, endurance and flexibility, while problems with vision and balance frequently occur; we become more vulnerable to extremes of temperature and have difficulties with fluid regulation. As well, there is a higher incidence of chronic disease in the elderly, and a greater susceptibility to infection. Some of these changes may ultimately prove to be preventable; certainly the effects of a number of them can be allayed by a sound diet and regular exercise. At present, though, the majority seem to be unavoidable; we have no choice but to learn to live with them.

The way that we garden will inevitably be affected as we grow older; but gardening itself brings many and varied benefits, some of which are quite apparent, while others may surprise. All make a contribution to our quality of life, and together can have a profound effect on the way in which we age.

Gardening as Physical Exercise

Perhaps the most obvious benefit of gardening is the exercise it provides—'use it or lose it' is an adage which contains much truth. In our society, ageing is generally associated with reduced physical activity. This is a real 'Catch 22' situation, for a good deal of the loss of function seen in the elderly is a consequence of a particular bodily part or system not being used. Disuse may be associated with joints becoming painful, or some temporarily debilitating disease. Bedrest itself can result in a general weakness that can make it more difficult to resume normal activities. This, in turn, means we miss out on the health benefits associated with the curtailed tasks—tasks such as a brisk walk to the shops, a stroll around the park, or a day at work in the garden. It is easy to see how, once started, this vicious cycle can fuel itself.

Exercise affects both our individual component parts and the way our overall system functions; it affects the bits we can see and bits we cannot. It is a powerful preventative for many of the less desirable aspects of ageing, able to arrest and in some cases reverse loss of function. Exercise benefits the elderly just as much as it benefits the young, and while a lifetime of physical jerks will stand us in good stead, benefits are gained even if we have never exercised before.

Exercise experts now recognise the contribution that everyday activities make to our physical fitness. As well as recommending some regular full-on exercise, modern exercise 'prescriptions' contain a component of these less demanding everyday exertions. Some of the more radical sport scientists are even of the opinion that we should *enjoy* our choice of exercise! Thus gardening is to be valued for its contribution to our own personal exercise programs. Unfortunately, it is this very aspect of gardening that causes many older gardeners to come unstuck, for it is in the physical demands of gardening that their difficulties lie.

Physical strength

Some loss of physical strength is seen as a normal part of the ageing process. Muscle strength peaks in our third decade, then it's downhill after that! It seems that the amount of muscle that we have as well as the strength of muscular contraction decreases as we grow older. Muscles do, however, respond readily to 'training' and those who have engaged in well designed muscle training programs throughout their adult lives may suffer little decline while these programs are maintained. Those of us whose 'weight training' has been of a more informal nature (lugging the laundry to the line, carting consumables from the car, or doing a day's digging on demand) are more likely to experience some losses. This loss of strength may be little more than a nuisance in itself, but it may lead to further problems by predisposing us to muscle strain by 'overdoing it', and may lead to more loss in function if it further downgrades our level of activity.

Forward planning is the key to successful gardening as we age, as with other areas of our post-retirement lives. There are several strategies we can adopt to deal with the effects of this loss of strength when gardening. We can:

1. Embark on a well-designed training program under the guidance of a professional. This may enable us to reverse the decline in strength to a degree and will stave off further losses. It must be stressed that the program should be conducted by someone with an understanding of both ageing and any specific medical problems we might have. All

of us *over forty-five* should seek the advice of a health professional such as a doctor or physiotherapist before commencing such a program.
2. Redesign our garden tasks so that they are appropriate to our physical capabilities.
3. Modify the garden environment to minimise the physical stress involved in working within it.
4. Invest in some specially designed tools that can be used to help to compensate for the effects of loss of strength when performing particular tasks.
5. Introduce warm-up exercises that can be done before gardening to ensure that we do not damage our muscles by working them while still cold.

These approaches are not, of course, mutually exclusive and any or all of them can be tried simultaneously. The choice of options will vary from one individual to the next—it will depend on our degree of disability, financial flexibility and personal disposition. While the option of the exercise program is beyond the scope of this book, the remaining aspects are dealt with in detail in later chapters.

Endurance

The cardiovascular system, that is, our heart and circulation, will undergo certain changes as we age. It seems that the actual constituent materials of the tissues are altered in a way that is regarded as part of normal ageing, with the result that many of us are unable to sustain demanding activities for as long as we previously could. However, our cardiovascular system, too, responds wonderfully well to training, and our heart and general circulation improves readily as we (carefully) increase our level of aerobic activities. 'Aerobic' here refers to anything that will raise the amount of oxygen that we burn up, and includes walking, swimming, jogging, and most exercise workouts.

These activities need not be high tech or done at a frantic pace to improve our health status; even something as apparently undemanding as bending and straightening the arms has proved useful as a daily workout for frail individuals who are chairbound. An elderly 'élite' athlete with a lifetime of training could well have a higher level of cardiovascular fitness than an untrained younger individual, and furthermore, low intensity exercise can improve our cardiovascular health at a similar rate to high intensity programs—the more 'aerobic' aspects of gardening have an excellent conditioning effect.

Heart disease remains the major cause of death world-wide for the over sixty-five age group. For individuals with cardiac complaints, gentle exercise may be the only form of exercise that is safe; everyday activities take on a particular importance as a means of physical exercise. Gardening can, to a large extent, be made as easy or strenuous as we choose. By careful design, gardening can provide us with our own custom-made exercise regime.

Heart disease often goes undetected until serious problems arise, and *everyone* over forty-five years of age should consult their doctors before initiating any change in their level of physical activity.

Osteoporosis

Osteoporosis is a common and frequently debilitating disease which affects mainly the elderly in our society. The loss of bone that is the hallmark of osteoporosis can lead to a loss in height and to curvature of the spine. Lower back pain is another symptom, caused by ultra-fine 'microfractures' of the backbone; these microfractures are also responsible for much of the disfiguration associated with the disease. Bones thinned by osteoporosis are easily broken and may fracture without any apparent trauma, such as a knock or a fall. Of course, a fall will do even more damage, and can be devastating to someone suffering from osteoporosis. When these fractures affect mobility, the consequences for our overall health care can be dire.

We reach our peak bone mass at around thirty years of age. After that, bone loss occurs gradually in both men and women, but increases abruptly in women after menopause. The first step in protecting ourselves against the disease is to make sure that we develop the best set of bones that we are capable of in the first place. While heredity has a large say in the matter, factors such as diet, exercise, smoking and alcohol consumption will all affect our skeletal health.

Load-bearing exercise such as walking, stair climbing, dancing and weight-lifting (but not swimming) will help us develop our bones to their maximum potential. Maximising and maintaining our skeletal well-being throughout adult life through an adequate diet and regular weight-bearing exercise will help offset the effects of later bone loss. The walking and moving, carrying and carting that are a normal part of gardening activity have a significant role to play in guarding us against the deleterious effects of osteoporosis.

Flexibility

Most of us will develop problems with our joints as we grow older. It seems that changes in the chemical components of the joints are an inevitable part of ageing: these changes prevent the components from performing their normal cushioning functions, causing pain and discomfort at the joint. Many of us will also develop joint disease; osteoarthritis in particular is extremely common in older people. Some eighty per cent of people over sixty-five will show signs of this disease, which is considered by some to be a universal part of normal ageing. Add to this the number of older people suffering from other forms of arthritis, and the loss of agility that we see in the elderly would seem to be explained.

However, again, disuse makes a contribution to joint stiffness, for an unused joint will soon 'seize up'. Those in need of convincing should take note that although elderly people are generally thought to be unable to perform fast, precise finger movements, many musicians perform perfectly well into old age. Arthur Rubinstein was still playing highly demanding Chopin piano concertos at eighty-eight, while André Segovia was giving concerts on classical guitar at ninety-two! While talent no doubt comes into it, it is the daily practice that is largely responsible for sustaining the expertise of these artists into advanced old age.

The effects of any training are highly specific—exercising one's left arm *will not* do a thing towards improving the right one—so we need to include a smorgasbord of activities in our daily routine. Gardening, with its combination of gross movement (walking, bending, reaching up and out) and fine control (planting out, taking cuttings, sowing seeds) is an excellent means of achieving the desired variety in movement modes, thus maximising our chances of retaining flexibility. However, those suffering from joint disease must take care not to aggravate the condition by overdoing things and a bit of a juggling act will be necessary to balance the benefits of exercise against the dangers of excess. The simple but often overlooked principle of pacing yourself is to be observed religiously in such cases: this will be dealt with in a later chapter.

Unavoidable Changes as We Age

Gardening as exercise can be of benefit in helping to overcome some of the problems that beset us as we age; this I find a most comforting thought. There are, however, age-related changes that do not respond to exercise. A number of these will affect us in the garden.

Changes in vision

There are some changes in our vision that will occur in all older individuals. The vast majority of us will need spectacles for reading, and while a good many will retain good long distance vision, some age-related changes in our eyesight will affect us in an outdoor environment.

The rate at which our eyes adjust to changes in light levels gradually lessens as we age; this means that it becomes more difficult for our eyes to cope with an abrupt change in illumination, thus either suddenly stepping into bright sunlight or entering deep shade can temporarily blind us.

Many older people, perhaps ten per cent over sixty years, experience Centre Field Loss of their eyesight. This results in their being able to only see things in the periphery of their vision while the image formed will be blurred and largely drained of colour. This reduction in colour vision is associated with an increased general sensitivity to light, experienced as 'glare'; cataracts too are highly light sensitive in their early stages of development. This heightened sensitivity to glare can prove problematic, especially if there are highly reflective surfaces, such as concrete or lightly coloured bricks. Difficulties in interpreting contrasts in colour and in light and darkness also arise, and can confuse our perception of depth.

These effects may seem inconsequential but in fact can be both disconcerting and distressing. More importantly though, all this can affect our safety in the garden. This is particularly so since changes in light are often associated with changes in levels or surfacing materials, for example, at the back door step or the decking under the pergola. An awareness of these changes helps to some extent but requires an unwavering concentration. Fine-tuning the garden environment is generally a far more reliable means of minimising these problems, ensuring maximum safety and security.

Falls

Older people are more likely to fall than their younger counterparts, and the consequences of a fall can be far more serious. The higher incidence of falls in older people can be due to changes in balance or vision, or to age-related hormonal disturbances or diseases of the nervous system. Most accidents in the home happen in transit areas such as garages, paths and patios, so attention to safety in these areas is vital where older people are concerned. Another cause of falls associated with ageing is the slower rate at which our blood pressure adjusts to a change in posture. Standing up too quickly can temporarily reduce the blood pressure in the brain, causing us to faint, and this should be taken into account when gardening.

Temperature regulation

Our temperature regulation also gets out of whack as we get older. Not only are our bodies slower to recognise the need to adjust to extremes of temperature, they are also less efficient at making the physiological adjustments that are needed to do so. This leaves us far more dependent on behavioural means of adjusting our body temperature, means such as putting on a jumper or moving into the shade. While hypothermia is unlikely to be a problem in the Australian climate, heat exhaustion is. Again, garden design should provide for this fact by incorporating shaded areas where they are needed. Our garden work plan should also take this into account by limiting the amount of time we spend working in the heat.

Damage from UV rays

Coupled with the problems of avoiding glare and heat stroke is our need to avoid excessive exposure to sunlight. Australia already has the dubious honour of having the highest incidence of skin cancer in the world, and the danger from the cancer-causing properties of ultraviolet light has of late been exacerbated by the holes in the atmospheric ozone layer. Our cellular repair mechanisms for UV damage decline as we age, making us far more at risk of developing skin cancer. More people are sunburnt in their own backyards than in any other venue, and both behavioural and design strategies should be employed to minimise this risk. 'Slip-Slop-Slap' by all means, but pay attention as well to layout; by thoughtful design of our garden environment we can help to avoid many of the less desirable consequences of growing older. These design issues are addressed in Chapter 5.

Horticulture as Therapy

Most of us will be at least vaguely aware of the therapeutic value of gardening. Some may quite consciously use it as a form of stress management or as an artistic pursuit. That gardening is used formally by health workers as both therapy and rehabilitation may nevertheless come as a bit of a surprise. Horticulture is used for people with a wide range of physical disabilities—road accident victims, people who have had strokes or heart attacks, amputees, people in wheelchairs or on walking frames, with the use of only one hand or with limited vision. It is used with the mentally retarded and with those with impaired memory, and is used as well in drug rehabilitation and with people suffering from emotional disorders. It is used, too, perhaps most poignantly, with our institutionalised elderly in hospitals and nursing homes. This focused use of gardening has helped to identify some of the less obvious ways that we benefit from gardening.

Gardending, it is said, benefits us on all levels—the physical, the intellectual and the emotional; some would add 'the spiritual'. While the non-physical benefits of gardening for older gardeners are difficult to measure, their effects are more easily observed.

Intellect and ageing

One factor that seems to be important in successful ageing is intellectual stimulation—'use it or lose it' is as true of our intellectual capabilities as it is for our physical functions. What is more, many people find on retiring that earlier curiosities are reawakened, leading to a rekindling of the desire to learn. That this is no uncommon thing can be seen in the success of organisations catering for this growth, organisations such as The University of the Third Age; even institutions like the Council for Adult Education who do not specifically cater for elders, find significant numbers of older people enrolling in their courses.

Of course, this appetite for learning may not always manifest itself in so formal a way. We have seen already how gardening often leads to the development of expertise in some aspect of horticulture. This may involve one particular group of plants, a single species of the garden wildlife, a particular style of garden design or the history of gardening itself; or it may encompass a little of each, and very much more besides. Though this may well occur through the scholarly pursuit of knowledge, it is just as likely to develop in a less structured way. In terms of personal growth and life satisfaction, their value is the same.

Stress and health

Stress has been shown to influence both the development and the outcome of a large number of life-threatening conditions such as heart disease, cancer and infectious diseases. Curiously, the amount of stress produced by a given event will vary from person to person, and what one experiences as mildly distressing another may find devastating. Those least affected are usually the people who have adequate 'coping strategies' for dealing with stressful events. Some lucky people seem to have a naturally easy-going disposition that allows them to cope with stress with no apparent effort, but in fact, most coping strategies are developed by trial and error over the years, either consciously or unconsciously.

There are a number of stressful life events that are more likely to occur in later life. These include the loss of a spouse, the moving away of a member of the family and the deterioration of some aspect of our health. Retirement itself is sometimes regarded as a negative life event. Many people put high value on the stress-reducing effect of gardening and many of us use it quite consciously as a means of unwinding. Some will find this calming effect in the garden environment itself: humankind evolved in a green landscape, a landscape that was full of challenges and dangers while yet affording some measure of comfort and safety. While these early associations may remain only in the subconscious, the resultant emotional responses are with us still. Other gardeners will find relief in the almost meditative state that active gardening can induce; others still will find it through the outlet that gardening provides for their aggressive feelings, perhaps in tilling the soil, chopping down an unwanted tree or yanking out the weeds—I can personally attest to the cathartic effects of a heavy prune!

Medical science is now confirming what for long has stood as common sense—that there are very real links between our emotional health and our susceptibility to disease. Happiness and peace of mind can have powerful effects on our physical well-being. Laughter, it has been found, is the best medicine *not* because it provides a distraction from our woes but because it enhances our immune responses. It does this through a pervasive chemical network that links our nervous system to our immune system and which 'conducts our orchestra of the immune system'. That we are less likely to fall ill when we are on a 'high' is a common experience. We may still have some distance to go before our understanding of the physiological consequences of our emotional states can explain the health-promoting effects of joyful experiences. Even so, the life-enhancing effect of gardening for the gardener is something few devotees would question.

Gardening as work

Much is made in the Horticultural Therapy literature of the value of gardening as a work substitute. While there will be those amongst us who will regard 'work' as a gardening substitute (no need to declare where I stand on that issue!), it seems clear that, as a species, we do have a need for productive activity of some kind. The statistics show that most of us adjust well to retirement; however, there are some who find the transition difficult, and it is perhaps these individuals for whom the 'work' aspect of gardening is most important. At any rate, the satisfaction of providing for some of our material needs is a very real one.

For those with a strong competitive streak, retirement from the workplace may rob them of an outlet for this. Although 'competition' may be a dirty word in some circles, it is deeply entrenched in many of us, and it is probably more realistic to accommodate it than to deny its importance. A competitive streak can be constructively employed in the garden, either formally through organised competitions (biggest pumpkin, best rose, most beautiful garden), or informally, by simply improving on our own previous efforts.

Formal Horticultural Therapy

Horticultural Therapy is used in some institutions such as prisons, rehabilitation centres and of course, nursing homes for the elderly. One of the most dehumanising aspects of life in an institution is the lack of control that 'inmates' have over their lives. This is just as true for older people as it is for their younger counterparts, and is something that few of us will have trouble empathising with. For the institutionalised elderly, the introduction of some form of active gardening offers them a chance to exercise control over some part of their environment, albeit only a tiny part. The fact that their efforts *matter* to some other living thing can have an enormous effect on self-esteem; the ongoingness and seasonality that are an inherent part of gardening can give shape and purpose to what is often a featureless existence. These restorative effects can occur whether the gardening involves a large productive garden, a small plot of flowers, or just a single potted plant at the bedside. The very large consequences of a very little gardening highlight some of the often unrecognised benefits that the activity offers.

So those of us who garden can congratulate ourselves on how clever we have been to have engaged in such a beneficial activity—for once, something we enjoy is not immoral, illegal or fattening! Those who are drawn to take up gardening, perhaps for the very first time, can do so assured it will be a tonic for the mind, body and soul—and a source of joy for the years to come.

2
People and Gardens

PEOPLE AND GARDENS GO BACK A LONG WAY. FROM THE BIBLICAL GARDEN of Eden to the legend of Shangri-la, we have placed The Garden fair in the centre of our paradise myths—to the collective human consciousness, a garden is as good as it gets! We have been making gardens, too, for a very long time, perhaps since the dawn of civilisation. It is the grand gardens of the past that have survived, in record or reality—the gardens of the Pharaohs, the towers of Babylon, Villa Lante, Versailles. While these gardens may inspire us and fire our imaginations, it is the gardens we make for ourselves that will be the most significant in our lives.

In Australia, almost forty per cent of the population garden as a form of recreation, while in the United States it is estimated that on any given weekend around three quarters of all American households will be out there working the earth; gardening has become a national pastime in more countries than our own. What is more, gardening is an activity which cuts across barriers of class, race and economics; so too is it enjoyed by women and men alike. While gardening crosses barriers of class, religion, race and gender, the likelihood that we will garden as a recreation increases as we age. Furthermore, most of us develop our gardening skills gradually over many years and it is in later life that we reach our full powers as gardeners.

It is often among older people that we find our most ardent gardeners: it is often among them, too, that we find the most remarkable. What follows are brief 'gardening portraits' of some remarkable older gardeners—they are a fascinating and inspiring lot. Some garden in the public eye, opening their gardens to all, while others are unheard of beyond their own small circles. Some garden in a way that seems untouched by their age, while some must overcome considerable pain or disability in order to do so. Their 'gardeners' tales' indicate how varied are the successful approaches to gardening as we age, for while a love of gardening is common to them all, their ways of gardening are as diverse as are their gardens.

Tom Garnett will be known to many gardeners on two counts. Firstly, as the gardening writer T. R. Garnett, he has educated, entertained and encouraged readers of the Melbourne newspaper *The Age* for over fifteen years. Though his thought-provoking articles centre around the garden, their topics often extend beyond the strictly horticultural; he sees the forest *and* the trees, placing gardening in both a personal and a cultural context.

Then, he will be known as co-creator of 'The Garden of St Erth' to the thousands of people who have visited the garden over the years. The garden is set in the hills of the Wombat State Forest an hour north-west of Melbourne, near the old goldmining township of Blackwood. Four hectares of cleared land surround a nineteenth century sandstone cottage, and there the Garnett family have made a varied and beautiful garden. They open the garden to the public every day throughout the year; despite its size and its public nature, it remains in essence a private family garden.

The making of the garden *and* Mr Garnett's career as a writer both began after he had officially retired. While the writing was an unforeseen development, the garden was not. The property at Blackwood was originally bought by the Garnetts as a place to spend their weekends and holiday breaks. When Mr Garnett retired in 1973 after years as a headmaster, the family moved to St Erth with the intention of making a large and challenging garden. The garden has evolved over the years, rather than having been pre-planned, but the strong lines of the basic garden structure give coherence and a classic beauty throughout.

T. R. Garnett has chronicled the making of the garden in his book *The Evolution of a Gardener*. Those familiar with his writings will know his interests to include the native flora, local history and environmental concerns as well as horticultural practices, garden history and the use of Australian plants in the garden. The local wildlife frequently features in his articles; birds in particular hold a special fascination for him. The Garden of St Erth reflects these interests. Care has gone into creating different microclimates to provide a wide range of plants with the often very different conditions they require. The Garden of St Erth holds the official Victorian Ornamental Plants Collection of *Cistus* (Rock Rose) species. Beds of Australian native plants and a flourishing orchard act as powerful bird attractants. The birds, though, have a totally un-jingoistic approach to food and habitat and will choose whatever suits from either native or exotic.

Tom Garnett came from a family where an interest in both gardening and natural history were taken for granted. He built his first garden (a rock garden) during his undergraduate years, then as a young bachelor teaching in central London, he set up a window box at his rooms to attract the birds. A rash of planter boxes soon appeared on window ledges along the street, an early hint at the educative role he was to assume with gardeners in his later years.

Mr Garnett's scholarly approach to the plants he grows contributes much to the personal satisfaction provided by the garden, for he is as much a natural historian as he is a gardener. The act of gardening is also a source of great pleasure to him. Arthritis has long been a problem, one which necessitated three hip replacements fifteen years ago. (He is possessed of no more than the usual number of hips—one hip had to be redone.) He now walks with the aid of a stick but nevertheless still manages to garden. His approach to coping with his disability is characteristically multifacetted: With equal consideration for the plants and their human caretakers, garden beds at St Erth are mulched against weed invasion and surface evaporation, thus minimising the need for routine maintenance. Then, Mr Garnett has a number of tools designed for easy use by older gardeners. These include a kneeling frame, a garden gripper and a 'swoe' (see photo 1). These last two are light, long-handled tools that enable the gardener to work comfortably from a standing position. The Garnetts have brought back a number of such tools from their visits to the UK, for there is a wider range of gardening tools available there than there is in Australia at present. He also uses a sit-on mower to do much of the mowing that this large garden requires. The lawn, incidentally, is present as much for its value as a fire-break as for its appearance. Finally, Tom Garnett has help where he needs it. His wife Penelope has always been an equal partner in this venture, and she still does an enormous amount in the garden. The scale of the garden as well as the high standard of maintenance that its public nature requires mean that additional outside help is also needed.

While Mr Garnett *can* imagine life without a garden, it would necessitate a complete change of life-style, along with new interests, perhaps coupled with living by the sea, or in the city. He points out that he has lived in the city as a young man, 'without' a garden; when reminded that he soon made a window garden for himself there, he says 'Ah, yes', and admits that, without a garden in his life, there would be a considerable gap to be filled!

**(*Author's note*: Since this was written, Mr Garnett's health has deteriorated, and he can no longer garden as he would like to at St Erth. The Garnetts have decided to hand St Erth over to gardening colleague Clive Blazey and move to a smaller garden in Castlemaine. He will continue to write about gardening, and is looking forward to growing things in pots.)

For some people, gardening is an intense creative experience; **Barbara Maund** is one such person. A passionate gardener since childhood, Mrs Maund has lived and gardened in Castlemaine for the past decade. The first of her two gardens in the district was opened to the public as part of the Victorian Open Garden Scheme, and has been recorded in photograph and text in *Private Gardens of Australia* by Sarah Guest. Her current garden, her second in the region, was begun in 1991 and has also been part of the Australian Open Garden Scheme. It is currently open to the public on the first Sunday of every month.

A lifetime of seeking 'quality' plants has made Mrs Maund a knowledgeable and discerning plantswoman. She has planned her garden using plants selected for their colour, form and fragrance as well as their suitability for the often harsh conditions of Central Victoria. The plantings combine flowering shrubs and herbaceous perennials; silver and bronze leaved foliage plants are used throughout.

While the beauty of the plants and the skillful use of colour may first draw one's attention, it is Mrs Maund's use of geometric form which gives this garden its distinctive character and leaves the most lasting impression. The slope of the quarter acre block necessitates some changes in level, and Mrs Maund has created a series of small terraced beds linked by gentle steps and gravelled paths, which are balanced and harmonised by her sense of overall proportion. The relationship between the shapes of the beds and the adjoining areas are as important, and as much of a source of delight, as the plants themselves. Barbara Maund consciously designs her gardens as 'a game for responsible people', to excite and revitalise; there is a wit and playfulness in this garden that is more usually associated with the fine arts. All this has been achieved on a very tight budget, the result of steadfastness of vision and purpose in the face of considerable financial constraints.

While it is in meeting the creative and horticultural challenges of the garden that her greatest satisfactions lie, Mrs Maund also values the physical exercise that gardening provides. Her sculptural approach and exacting standards mean that there is always something in need of attention. Much time is spent on cutting back and in moving or replacing

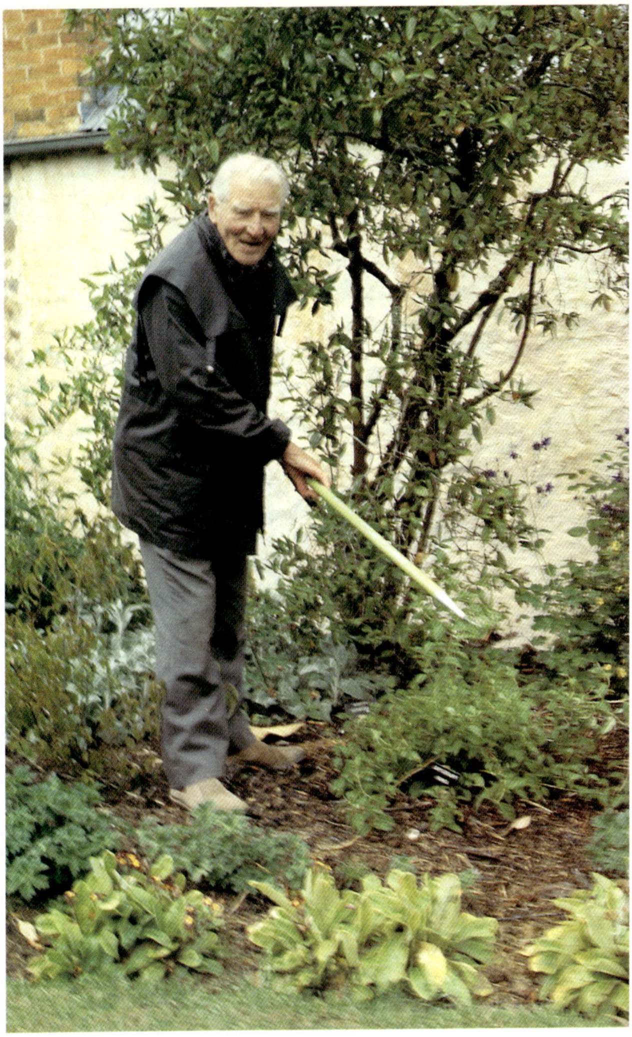

Tom Garnett *in action with his swoe*

1

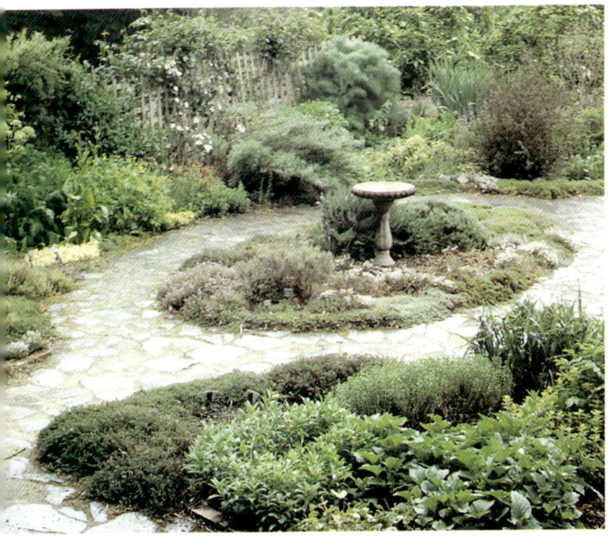

erb garden at St Erth 2

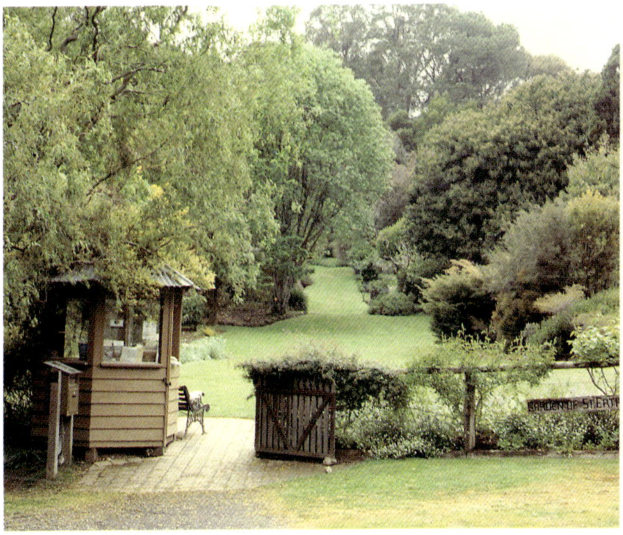

The entrance to the Garden of St Erth 3

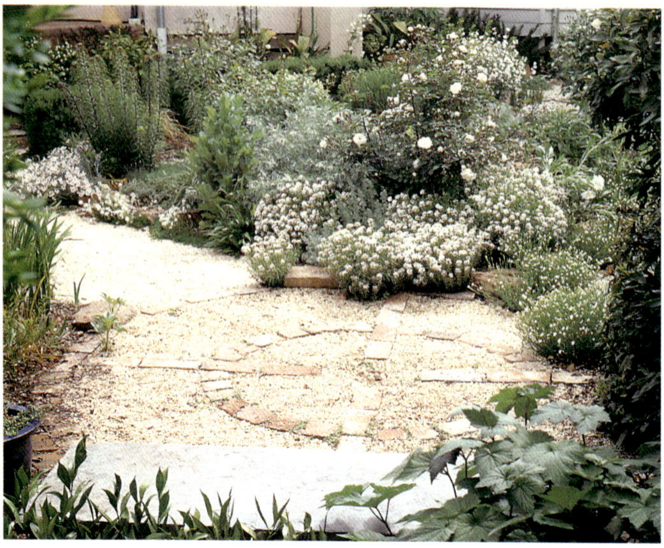

The white corner in Barbara Maund's garden 4

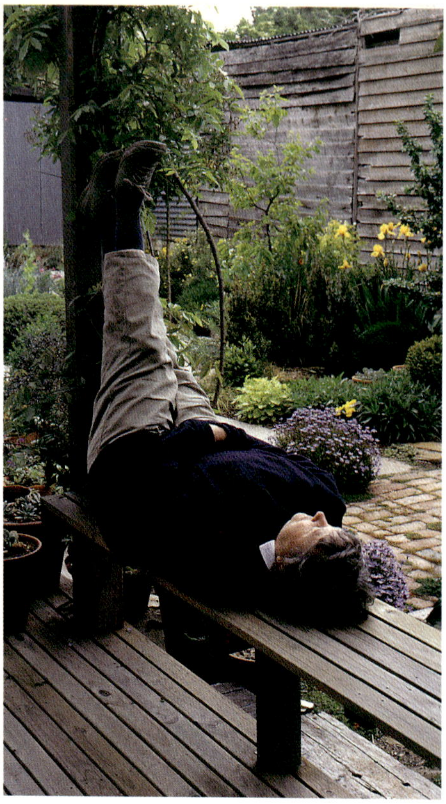

Right: Barbara Maund *taking a well-earned rest* 5

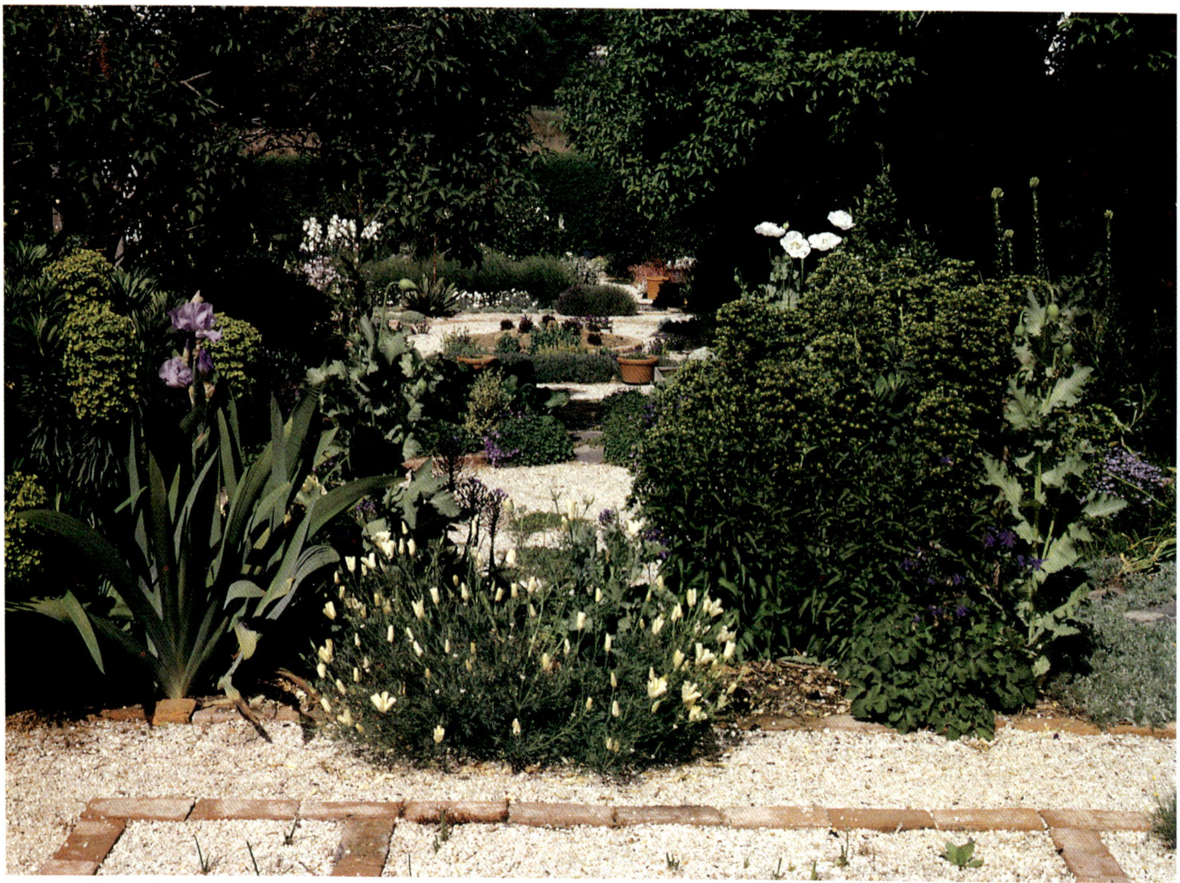

A view down the terraces in the Maund garden 6

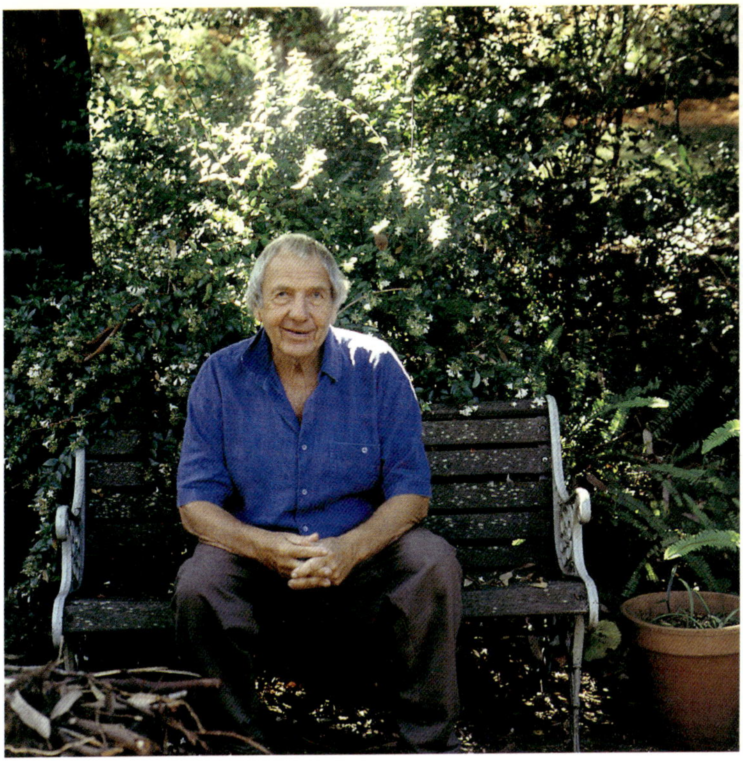

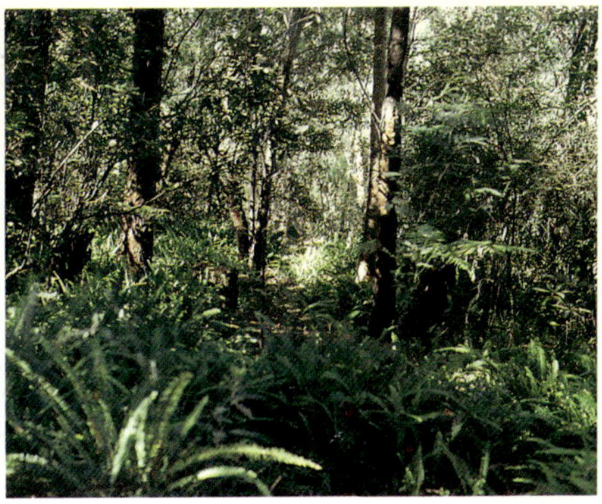

7

The bushland Gordon Ford *has created over the past four decades.*

Left: Gordon Ford *in his bush garden*

8

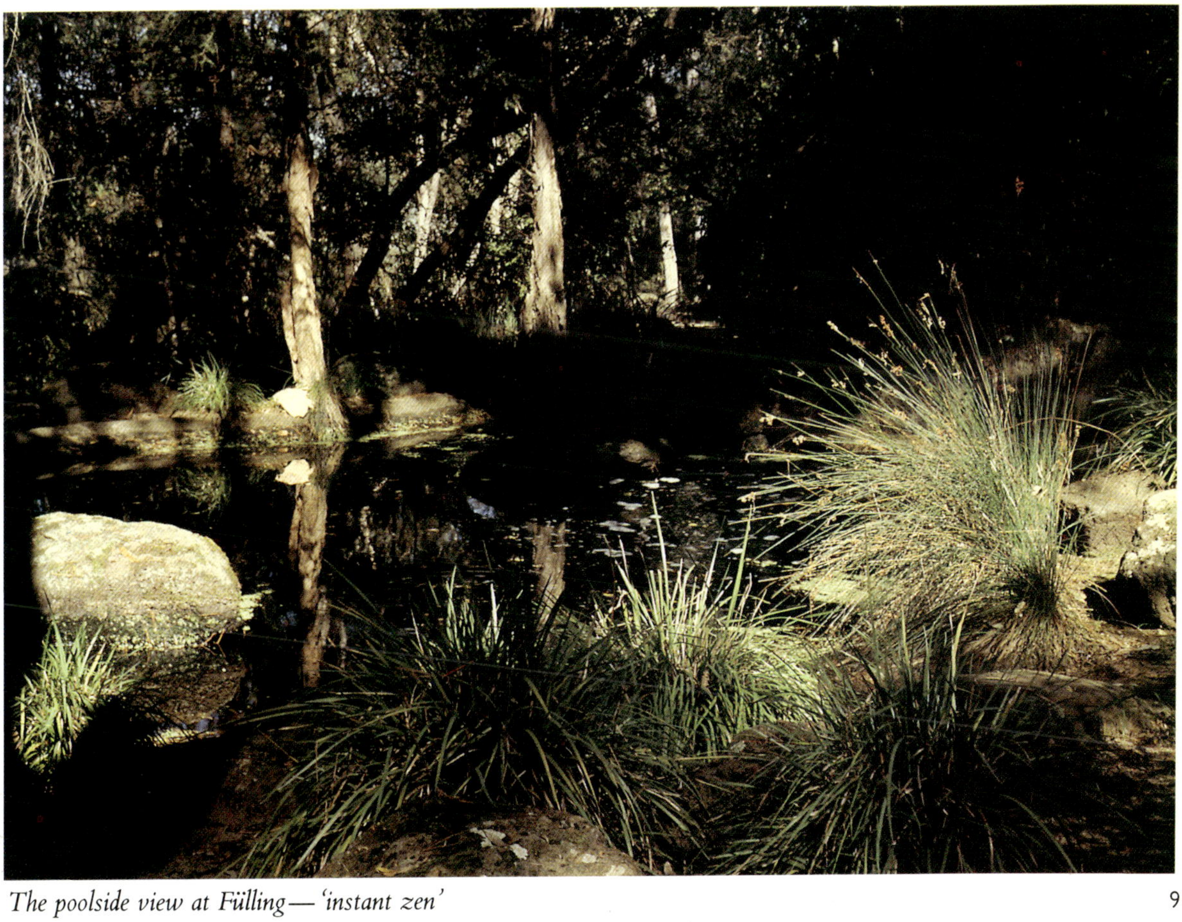

The poolside view at Fülling — 'instant zen'

9

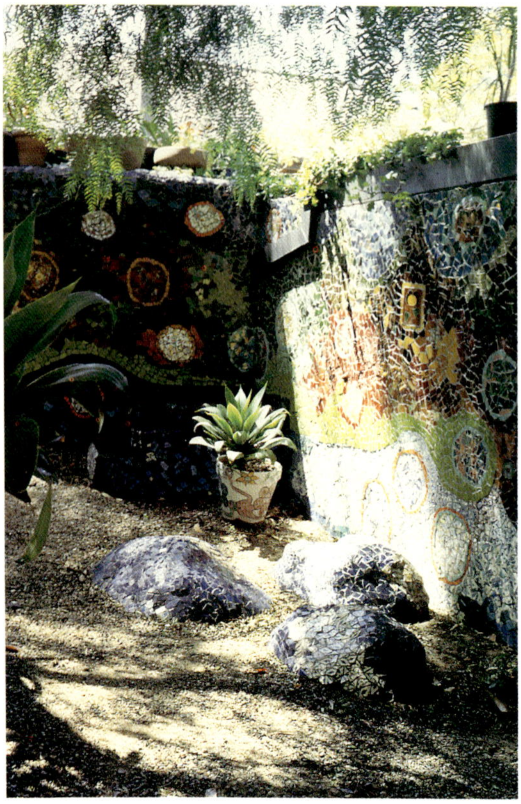

A sunlit corner of the Mosaic Garden 10

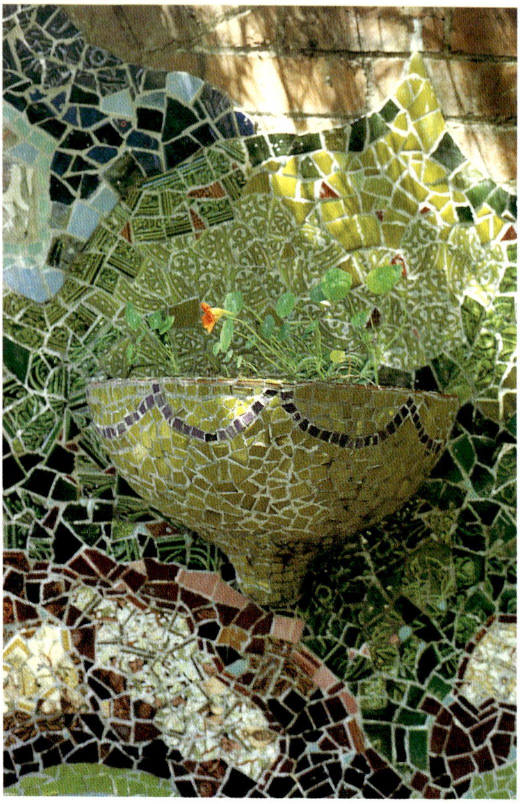

A delicate mosaic wall planter 11

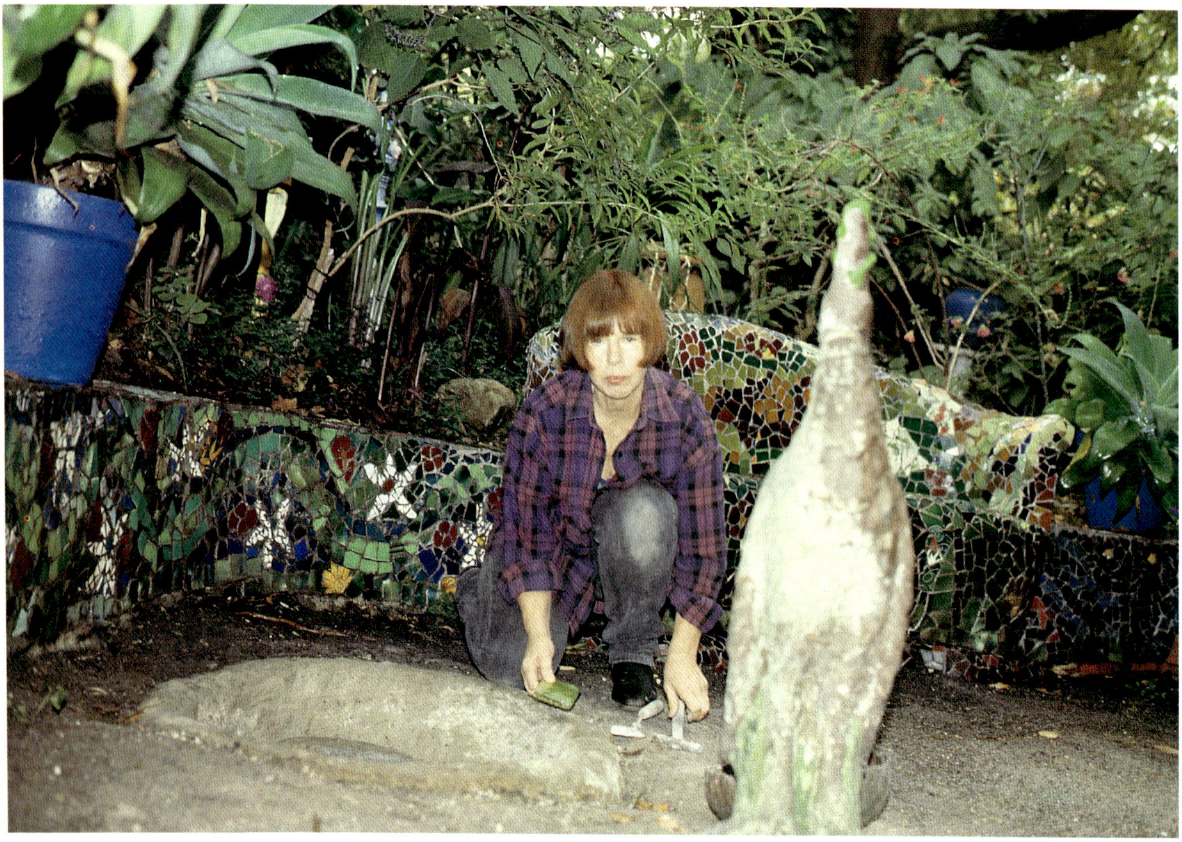

Margot Knox *at work on her Mosaic Garden* 12

plants that are past their best, or perhaps not up to par. She also has a somewhat unusual enthusiasm for weeding. There are no lawns to maintain but Mrs Maund has the large hedge of English Box along the front boundary clipped professionally as needed.

Mrs Maund has a recurrent problem with one of her feet and is aware that she will not always be able to garden at her current pitch. She anticipates a design solution to this problem in which her current plantings will be replaced by less demanding 'structural' plants such as dwarf box shaped into domes and hedges, and dwarf cotoneasters. Rather than viewing this as a defeat, Barbara Maund looks forward with obvious excitement to this future 'architectural' garden. While Barbara Maund can contemplate life without a garden, it is only in the knowledge that there are other people's gardens and their gardening joys to share.

While for some people, garden-making is the major creative outlet in their lives, for others, it is one of several strings to their creative bows. Artist **Margot Knox** lives and gardens in a converted church in an inner urban area. The house occupies a large part of the corner block, but the presence of the garden is felt strongly throughout. Views of the garden are framed by large windows all along one side, and tall glass doors stand open, leaving few barriers between outside and in. A shaded courtyard serves as the family dining-room in all but the wildest weathers, and is Mediterranean in both function and feel. The whole is enclosed by a high brick wall which marks the boundary between this most singular garden and the mundane outer world.

The front garden is separate from, and very different to, the side garden; it is in the front garden that the presence of Margot's muse is most strongly felt. This, the Mosaic Garden, is lush, rich, wild, exotic, beautiful though startling, and very, very, 'female'. Growing in spirit from the agaves that are the nucleus around which the garden crystallised, this garden is mysterious and filled with many treasures. Margot's sculpted garden forms are bold and organic, their blunt shapes bejewelled by a mosaic of broken ceramics.

A small and dainty woman in her sixties, Margot Knox has done all the hard landscaping herself. Since moving there eight years ago, she has rebuilt one wall, put in seats, ponds, retaining walls and paving. She explains that she acquired her skills while working with the innovative Australian bush gardener and stonemason Ellis Stones during the 1950s. Stones felt that women were often more 'sympathetic' stoneworkers than men, and this proved to be the case with Margot. Despite the hard labour involved, she soon became a skillful and efficient stoneworker, finding particular success as a paver.

Margot had grown up in a family where 'survival gardening' prevailed. She, however, was always 'a bit dreamy' about gardens, with a taste that ran more to overgrown cottages than vegetable patches. Margot started her first garden as a young woman when she and her late husband, architect Alistair Knox, built their first home in Eltham. Alistair wanted a native garden and Margot was restricted to the vegetable garden though she included flowers in this as an outlet for her more romantic garden leanings. Two houses later, their home sported both a native garden and a large kitchen garden, with a vegetable patch, fruit trees and roses.

Parallel to her garden-making runs Margot's painting. In the past, this has been her main artistic outlet and is still a major part of her creative life. Of late, she says, in common, with many of her similarly aged friends, the garden has become a passion, and has come to take up more and more of her life. In both her painting and garden-making, Margot finds she has become braver, more disciplined, less willing to compromise as she grows older. A landscape painter since early adulthood, she has now begun to paint the personalised landscapes of private gardens. Her annual exhibition this year will hold, for the first time, portraits of gardens and their gardeners. These exhibitions are held in her home, when she opens both her home and her garden to the public.

Margot is an inveterate planter. She sprinkles seeds along the lanes and alleyways near her home, seeding cracks between the cobbles wherever the chance presents. She claims that she is not a particularly skillful horticulturist, but delights in making something from nothing and is at her most inventive when her resources are limited. She is drawn to work on her garden each day, and spends much time thinking about her garden while not actively working in it. Margot is strong and nimble, but with its raised beds, general mulch, and paved and shady courtyard, maintaining the garden would be within the capabilities of a much less able-bodied gardener.

As well as her home garden, Margot has an allotment in a local community garden. There, she grows the annual crops that she has no room for at home. This summer, she and her children grew an abundance of herbs and sunflowers, and row after row of zinnias. These she stacked in bowls and vases throughout the house, their splendid bounty filling every available space throughout the season.

Life without a garden is inconceivable to Margot; she will always garden, even if she has nought but a balcony on which to carry out her schemes. She hopes that, when she dies, she'll go out pushing a wheelbarrow!

A sense of spiritual renewal is often experienced by gardeners when working or simply *being* in their gardens. When this sense is combined with a professional involvement in garden-making, the result is fortunate for all concerned.

Gordon Ford is a landscape designer who has been making Australian bush gardens in and around Melbourne for the last forty years. He has been a force in the evolution of the bush garden as we know it, pioneering the use of Australian plants in his gardens both for their visual properties and their suitability for the physical environment. His gardens are carefully composed works of asymmetrical balance where both living and non-living components are of equal importance. Rock work, land forms, water and plants are used to sculpt a garden where 'mass and void', shape and texture, light and shade, are finally the prime garden elements.

Mr Ford had no formal training in either landscaping or horticulture, but rather came to garden-making after working for Ellis Stones in the early 1950s. He took to landscaping immediately and it became his life's work. Prior to this, his only experience with gardening had been as a child, when he would sometimes help his mother in her cottage-style garden; later, as a public servant for the Forests Commission, he learnt about Australian trees. He then attended classes run by Ernest Lord (author of *Trees and Shrubs for Australian Gardens*), so building on his earlier informal horticultural education. Gordon Ford's approach to landscaping is both as a designer and a philosopher. He perceives garden-making as recreating 'the paradise within', naming the bushland of NSW in which he spent his childhood as the force that shaped his personal vision of paradise. He began creating gardens in his own particular style quite intuitively, with little understanding of why they 'worked'. He discovered later that the principles he had instinctively employed had been used by the English Landscape Movement of the eighteenth century, and by Japanese garden designers across the ages. He now uses these principles quite consciously and has further absorbed these styles in the development of his current garden ethos.

His own private garden, 'Fülling', is a bushland oasis in a suburb on Melbourne's northern fringe. Opening to the public as part of the Australian Open Garden Scheme, it is both beautiful and tranquil. Originally the block had been covered in bush, but this was cleared to make way for an orchard at the turn of the century. The orchard, in turn, was cleared and subdivided for a housing development after the war. When Gordon Ford bought the land in 1945, few trees remained and shrubby regrowth had established itself with great tenacity throughout the one and a half acre block.

Parts of the garden have been designed to spend time in and take in at some length, while others are designed to be passed through; seats are set largely in clearings, though some are placed within the bush. A narrow path winds through the trees, affording glimpses of sunlit glades and ferned gullies; low growing shrubs and grasses draw the eye to the bush floor.

This bush floor has been built up over the years by continuous mulching until the overhead canopy was established. Five hundred cubic metres of wood chips went into mulching the original plantings, all of it moved by hand. Now it is largely self-maintaining, with only the odd spot of weed removal and the occasional top up of wood shavings to supplement the leaf litter from the now mature trees.

The house is reached by stepping stones across a pool fed by a waterfall. There is a paved area adjacent to the pool, with a brazier to warm the chilly nights. Nearby is a bench overlooking the pool; here Gordon plants himself for 'instant Zen' when he feels the need. At seventy-five, he still works full time and has no plans of retiring.

Landscaping is much more than just a job to Gordon Ford. Creating gardens is still a joy to him, one which is central to both his professional and personal life; he could not live without a garden. He quotes the following passage to give voice to his feelings for his wild bush garden:

> And this our life, exempt from public haunt,
> Finds tongues in trees, books in running brooks,
> Sermons in stones, and good in everything.
>
> W. Shakespeare, *As You Like It*, act 2, scene 1.

Herbert Stanley **'Steve' Stevenson** and his wife Dorothy have lived and gardened in their bayside Melbourne home for over fifty years. The region was once a market garden area, and Dorothy's grandfather was amongst the first market gardeners in the district, setting up his enterprise in 1854 in what was then a recently drained swamp. The market garden was passed on from father to son for five generations until the whole area was converted to a giant shopping complex.

Steve Stevenson grew up in a household where both parents gardened, but in an unusual bit of role reversal,* his father cared only for growing flowers and trees, his mother only for 'useful' plants. They lived on the city outskirts to the north of Melbourne, and the family had only a single tank for their water supply; each summer would see a battle for the salvaged household wash water, with Father's ornamentals vying with Mother and the vegie patch for the rights to the recycled water.

When Mr Stevenson was seven, his father had a motorbike accident; Mr Stevenson Snr was unable to work for several years, and young Steve was sent to live in rural Victoria with his maternal grandparents. Steve loved living in the country and being part of the extended family that was the Hamilton of those days. His grandparents lived on an acre or so of land, and his grandfather had a beautiful vegetable garden and a small orchard with multiple-graft fruit trees, all in main view of the house. Steve spent many happy hours helping his grandfather in the garden, or accompanying him when he visited local Chinese market gardeners for

---

* Author's note: This is not lightly said. While there is little difference in the numbers of men and women who garden, there is notable difference in the way the two sexes garden.

the vegetables that Grandad did not grow. To this day, Mr Stevenson remembers and even practises some of his grandfather's tricks, such as first scattering his bean seeds on top of the soil and planting them only after they begin to sprout.

Steve returned to his parents' home when he was fourteen and was soon apprenticed as a trainee engineer. This was not a happy time for him; he missed the country life very much and longed to move back to Hamilton. Though proud of his trade, he has never found it easy working in a factory, cooped up all day with the noise and the smells; as a young apprentice, he told his uncomprehending father: 'If God made man and woman, he made them in a garden, not a factory!' When Steve married at twenty-one, he found relief from his factory life in a garden of his own, tending it every evening on his return.

Fruit trees and vegetables have always been Mr Stevenson's main interests; while he may have acquired his enthusiasm for productive gardening from his grandfather, it was his market gardening father-in-law who supplied him with both practical assistance and tools for this first garden. Steve's skills as an engineer soon led to him making his own gardening tools, improving on designs used by the market gardeners, modifying them to suit his individual needs; fifty years down the track, he is still using the tools he has made, and making new ones when the need arises.

In the front of the Stevensons' quarter acre block there is a garden of largely native trees with an understorey of shrubs and ferns; this has been consciously developed as a high-shade low maintenance area. A childhood without mains water has made water conservation an issue for Mr Stevenson, and the garden is mulched throughout; leaf litter and a living mulch of fish-bone ferns cover the ground in the front garden, isolated fruit trees are mulched with bricks while the vegetable patch is mulched in straw.

The vegetable garden is raised not to improve access but to allow regular additions of organic matter to the light sandy soil. However, the tools that Steve Stevenson has made for his own use are all small and long-handled, and he can do almost all his work from a standing position by the side of the beds. The exceptions to this are sowing seed and planting out seedlings; though generally hale and hearty, he has difficulty getting up and down from a kneeling position, and uses a kneeling frame to help him with this.

Mr Stevenson enjoys experimenting with different gardening techniques and reads widely on horticultural methods. Over the last twenty years or so he has developed an interest in medicinal herbs and companion planting and grows many such plants along side his crops. While his main interest has always revolved around productive gardening, his relationship with his plants is not a straight forward one of simply valuing them for their usefulness; he is especially proud of his culture of French Dandelions, but refuses to dig them up in order to make the dandelion coffee that he loves—instead, he buys the powdered roots from the local health food store!

Steve Stevenson cannot imagine life without a garden. He still dreams of moving to the country; untouched by his wife's admonishments that he is too old to move, he reasons that since he has so much *fun* with his current small block, he could have even more with a big one!

Food gardens were once an important part of all households with access to land enough to plant one. Today, food production techniques may have removed the need to grow our own food for survival but the importance of productive gardens remains for many gardeners.

Mary Watson has lived and gardened at the same address for nearly sixty years. Over that time she has developed a large and productive food garden behind her modest Edwardian home in a south-eastern Melbourne suburb. She established the garden soon after moving there as a bride and it comes as a surprise to learn that Mrs Watson's only previous gardening experience came when, as a schoolgirl, she took part in a school competition to grow the biggest radish; Mary Watson won first prize. Her parents did not garden but a lack of gardening background proved no disadvantage and young Mrs Watson soon had a flourishing food garden supplying more than enough for the needs of her young family.

Today the garden still boasts a large vegetable patch and a number of fruit trees including apple, peach, pear and apricot. Last winter she had a plum and a fig tree removed because they were interfering with her two avocado trees. These avocados are Mary Watson's pride and joy. One she grew from the seed of the first avocado she had ever tasted; this seedling did not bear fruit for the first ten years of its life. The second tree is grafted, a gift from a friend who knew of her impatience with the first one. Fifteen years on, the trees provide her with an almost continuous supply of avocados throughout the year.

Mary Watson comes of doughty stock. Her great-great-grandmother sailed to Australia from England in the hope of a better life; she came in the company of her eight children following the death of her husband. She and her children settled in Bendigo in central Victoria after travelling there largely on foot from their landing place, said to have been somewhere in South Australia. The following century her great-great-granddaughter Mary was born three miles outside of Bendigo. Mary weighed less than a kilo at birth and was not expected to survive. However, survive she did, to spend the first six months of her life wrapped in cottonwool, so small her mother swore the tiny babe would fit inside a gentleman's coat pocket. Now eighty-five years old, Mary Watson is still surprising people.

Mrs Watson has had no formal instruction in gardening, nor has she ever gone to books for information, but has learnt almost entirely by her own experience. An exception to this is her skill in grafting fruit trees; this she was taught by a friend. Many of her fruit trees sport multiple grafts. Her current exhibition pieces are two multiply grafted apple trees. One, a free-standing Red Granny Smith has been grafted with Jonathan, Red and Golden Delicious, and Granny Smith, to name but a few. Mrs Watson has espaliered the second apple tree against a low wire support. There is a different range of apples on this tree, including ten as yet unidentified varieties she was given last winter and which she grafted, as always, on the second week of August. These most recent grafts are bearing fruit already in this, their first season, and the identification of these newcomers should soon be possible.

She has trained these two apple trees into low-growing, compact shapes; she realised the value of doing so when she could no longer harvest the fruit from the upper branches of her other trees. Fortunately, as Mrs Watson had long grown more than enough for her own needs, she had already developed a 'skill-share' system with friends and neighbours and those who help harvest the fruit may keep half of their pickings.

Mary Watson loves to garden just as much as she ever did. She grows all her vegetables from seeds she has saved from previous years, often finding hybrids amongst the different strains she has grown: experimentation and discovery are still important components in her gardening. Although unable to garden for as long as she once did, she still spends hours at a time working there—'When I get out in the garden the time just flies!'

An arthritic hip restricted her movement at one stage, but after a successful hip replacement ten years ago, a determined Mrs Watson was gardening and riding her bike just six weeks after the operation. Nowadays she has trouble bending but the problems this creates are minimised by her long-standing use of tools that allow her to garden while standing up. Among her collection of small, long-handled tools, her favourite is a weeder-cum-hoe made for her by her late husband from a metal shelf bracket and a broom handle. Since her hip replacement she has acquired a kneeling frame and uses this whenever she has to kneel.

Mary Watson cannot imagine what life would be like without her garden. Her often serendipitous adaptations for gardening in retirement mean she may never need to find out.

3
Enabling Tools

TOOLS ARE OFTEN THE MEANS BY WHICH WE ADAPT TO GARDENING IN later life. Tools which allow us to work in a comfortable position, which do not cause strain simply by their use, will make a difference to any gardener; where a gardener has a disability, appropriate tools may make gardening possible where it was not possible before.

Many of the tools that we use in the garden have been around for hundreds of years. Developed over the course of our long agricultural history, some have changed little over this time. Traditional in design and the materials from which they are made, there is something deeply satisfying about the way they feel, the way they handle. Many perform their intended tasks superbly in the hands of their intended users, but therein can lie a problem, for their original users were often a far cry from the users of today.

These tools were largely designed for use by burly farm workers and are simply bigger and heavier than they need to be for today's home gardener. A garden implement of the seventeenth century was described by a writer of the time as 'sharp on both sides, which a man, with violence, thrusts before him'. Its user would undoubtedly have been a young man, conditioned by a life of hard physical labour and severe circumstance, for such heavy work fell usually to the men, and life was both harsh and brief: in the UK at this time, the average life expectancy for a male was probably around forty years, while in Roman times it was thirty-two. Today, the average life expectancy for a man in Australia is seventy-three years, while a woman can expect to reach almost eighty.

The Industrial Revolution saw the mechanisation of agriculture and the mass exodus of people from rural areas into the cities. Since then, there has been little need to work the fields with hand-drawn tools, and few people have more than a small space in which to garden. Women are no less likely than men to be actively involved in the garden, and furthermore, we grow more well disposed towards gardening as we grow older. The tools which have served the past generations well are not always the most appropriate for today's home gardener. The tools of yester-year were fashioned in the forge of the village blacksmith, and limited by the materials and the expertise at his avail. The development of new metal alloys along with the advent of modern manufacturing techniques have removed many of these restrictions. Recent technological advances have made it possible for tools to be made to virtually any shape and still be light and strong.

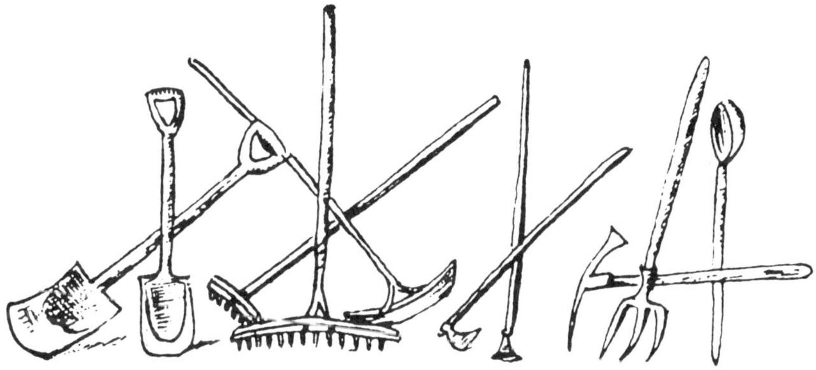

Garden tools of the early seventeenth century.

Wooden handles were, and still are, commonly attached to metal work-heads in our tools. Wood has many virtues: if chosen well, it is strong, it is light, it is pleasing to the touch; however, timber places limitations on the form of the handles that can be usefully fashioned. Trees are straight, but people not entirely so, and there are times when a handle of an unconventional shape will suit us better than a more commonplace version.

Ergonomics, the study of people at work, has given us some insight into what makes a tool a *good tool.* We work most efficiently when we are utilising the middle part of our range of strength and of our range of movement. As we grow older, both our strength and mobility become a little less than they were, and we need to adjust our choice of tools accordingly. Tools that are small and light are easier to hold, easier to use; there is less resistance to them as we move them through the soil, lift them through the air, pass them through the wood. Tools on long handles will allow us to work comfortably from a standing position, short-handled tools can be used when kneeling on a kneeling frame, while tools with handles of an intermediate length can be used while the gardener is seated. Finding the most comfortable working position and the best tools for these positions are important first steps in adjusting to our changing needs in the garden.

Beyond these first steps, though, there is more; again we can look to lessons learnt in the workplace for guidance. Every year, thousands of work-hours are lost around the globe due to the debilitating effects of Repetitive Strain Injury (RSI). The modern typist's equivalent of Tennis Elbow shows clearly that an action need not involve a lot of force in order to result in serious injury; even the lightest of actions performed in the best designed work station can cause considerable damage when repeated too many times over too long a period. What this means to us as gardeners is that we must plan our gardening to avoid staying at any one task too long, varying each activity with another that uses a different action or a different set of muscles. Workplace injuries have also highlighted the necessity for good posture and good lifting and carrying techniques. They have also shown the wisdom of knowing one's limitations and pacing oneself accordingly. All this we should take to the garden.

Tools Generally

Tool preference is a highly individual affair. What tools we find best to work with will depend on a number of factors, such as the position we like to work in, our physical strength, the soil we have to work with, as well as our little personal quirks in the way we like to garden. If we have been gardening for some time, our tool choices may depend less on these factors than on what we already have in the garden shed; it is important to look as critically at the tools that you already have as you would at any tools you were thinking of buying.

It is not only older gardeners who benefit from careful tool selection. Most of us will, at some stage, experience some form of temporary disability which will make it necessary for us to rethink the way that we do everyday things. We may have sprained an ankle, broken an arm, been pregnant, had to deal with things with an arm full of small child; whatever the cause, we will have found it necessary to find alternative ways of doing a number of necessary functions, sometimes for quite extended periods. Backache is particularly prevalent in our society—some eighty-five per cent of Australians will consult a doctor about back problems at some stage of their lives, many of them as relatively young adults. Our earlier ignorance of the importance of back care has meant that many an individual must spend their lives unable to lift or bend in the way that most of us take for granted; the consequences of a moment's forgetfulness can be days, even weeks, of severe pain, or even permanent disability. It has become necessary for many of us to reassess the way we go about our daily tasks, including the way we garden.

First Things First

Perhaps the first thing that we need to consider when choosing garden tools is the position that suits us best when working in the garden. If you find that bending a certain part of you is painful, or if you have been advised against doing so, then this may make your choices clear. However, there is sometimes a fine line to tread between 'use it or lose it' and avoiding the uncomfortable. Bending in the garden may be a valuable form of exercise, but it is somewhat unpredictable in its nature. It is important that we use all our joints and muscles as much as possible to keep them in good working order, however, it may be wiser to limit the use of a painful joint when gardening and substitute a more controlled form of exercise. If in any doubt, consult a health professional; your own doctor should be your first stop, then a physiotherapist or an occupational therapist for specialist advice. Occupational therapists, in particular, have a working knowledge of aids and gadgets; regional hospitals and community health centres normally have an occupational therapist on their staff, and your doctor can usually refer you to one on request. If you are already under care for a problem, be sure to check with the relevant authority before ringing in any changes, and make sure you comply with any existing orders on lifting, posture and so forth.

The next, and equally important, thing we need to consider is the size and weight of tools that suit us best. The smaller and lighter a tool is, the less strain it will cause to its user. A small tool will encounter less resistance from the earth, the plant, the water, and will be easier to lift if loaded up with leaves, soil or weedings.

Tool Sources

Many gardeners think no further than the local hardware store when it comes to buying tools. While useful tools can be obtained from these outlets, there are other less well-known ways of obtaining tools that are perhaps more likely to yield up the tools that we need. What follows is a brief run-down of where such tools can be obtained. The tools themselves are described more fully later in this section.

Mainstream retailers

There are, at present, only a limited number of lightweight tools commercially available. Most of the local tool companies make small handtools such as trowels and two-pronged weeders that have short handles, but amongst their longer-handled tools there are usually only one or two that are genuinely small and light. These are often sold as 'Ladies' or 'Campers' tools (forks or spades) and usually come in only one choice of handle length.

Amongst the most useful tools to be found through retail outlets such as hardware stores and garden centres is an imported range that features a large number of small, light tool-heads that attach interchangeably to handles of various lengths. Tool-heads are available to serve many different purposes, and the various handle lengths mean that the tools can be used from a standing, sitting, or kneeling position.

Rehabilitation suppliers

Another source of ready-made tools is medical rehabilitation suppliers. These companies do their main trade in items such as wheelchairs, ramps, shower rails and pick-up sticks, but in addition some stock a small range of garden tools designed for people with health problems or a disability. They may also have a range of auxiliary handles and extender devices for those gardeners who have problems gripping conventional tools. These companies can sometimes be hard to trace and may change from time to time, but can be located through your State Independent Living Centre (ILC) or through the occupational therapist at your local hospital or community health centre.

Although I have listed some of the main rehabilitation suppliers at the back of this book, it is a good idea to check with your State ILC to be sure that this information is still current. The ILCs not only carry a list of stockists, they also have a number of tools at their centres for people to look at. They assess all the equipment that comes their way, and if an item meets with their approval, they compile a fact sheet on the item which includes a description, measurements, benefits and drawbacks and who it is likely to suit; these sheets also list the stockists and the recommended retail prices at the time that the assessment was done. The staff of occupational therapists and other health workers at the ILC can advise people on what tools may suit them. This service is currently free to pensioners, but there is a *small* fee for others. (See the listings at the end of the book for the addresses of your State ILC.)

Private inventors

From time to time, an individual gardener will feel the need to improve upon existing garden tools, or even invent an entirely new one. Sometimes these designers turn out a tool that excites such a positive reaction from people that they go on to manufacture them. Such tools include the *Garden Gillie* and the *Ergonomic Shovel*, both of which I have described in this chapter. As yet, there is no official registry for these tools, and unless these small inventor-manufacturers can afford to pay for costly advertising (which they seldom can), or else manage to get some media exposure through life-style television programs or the gardening press (which does occasionally happen), many of these tools will remain unknown to the general gardening public. Most sell their tools only by mail order, running their businesses from their homes.

Some of these tools can be located through the State Independent Living Centres; the Horticultural Therapy associations in Victoria and NSW, and the Banksia Centre in the ACT may also be able to help with this. As well, Victorians have the good fortune of having the country's only 'Occupational Therapist—Horticulture', and she will advise on tools and garden design for those with a disability. These addresses are listed at the end of the book.

Modifying conventional tools or making your own

Another way of obtaining useful tools is by making them oneself or by modifying manufactured tools. In the days when garden tools were made by the village blacksmith, individual variations were easily incorporated into the designs. The Industrial Revolution saw the end of personalised tools and even of the local variations that were once the norm; mass production now gives us standardised tool designs almost across the board. Still, by modifying what the manufacturers choose to send our way, tools can be tailor-made to suit the needs of the gardener. Handles can be lengthened or shortened, grips built up, work-heads filed down to give a smaller, lighter tool.

If you are not 'handy' yourself, some smaller businesses such as hardware stores or mower shops (places you might go to, to have your pruners sharpened) can sometimes be prevailed upon to carry out these modifications for a small fee. Perhaps you have a 'dream tool' that does not exist; think about what features you would like to see incorporated into the tool; when you are clear about what you would like—tool-head, handle length, any additional grips—then you are ready to take the design to someone who might help you. There are also various 'add-on' devices that allow a tool to be gripped more firmly or used more easily. These I have described later in the chapter; they can be an effective and convenient way of making a tool more user-friendly.

Organisations to aid the disabled

There are organisations throughout Australia which run a wonderful service in making or adapting tools and aids for the disabled, when there is no commercial product or service available. Known as Technical Aid for the Disabled (TAD), they have branches in all capital cities; their numbers are given in the back of the book. Most of the city branches also have regional sub-branches. If there is an Independent Living Centre in your State, you should ring them *before* you contact your local TAD Branch, and they will give you the details of any commercially available option. TAD's clients have all types of disabilities and cover all age groups. Clients are often referred to them by a health professional such as an occupational therapist, physiotherapist or doctor, but people can refer themselves.

There is no charge for the TAD service. Volunteers give their technical skills free of charge, and clients are asked only to reimburse volunteers for any cost of materials and their travelling expenses.

The modifications they undertake are diverse and have included lengthening tools, raising equipment such as kneeling frames, and modifying equipment to allow its use by gardeners who can use only one arm or who are confined to a wheelchair. Below is a working diagram for lengthening the handle of a spade made for a client by a TADVIC (the Victorian branch) volunteer. It is an effective and secure way of extending tool handles. It is also quite simple, and within the capabilities of most 'handy' individuals.

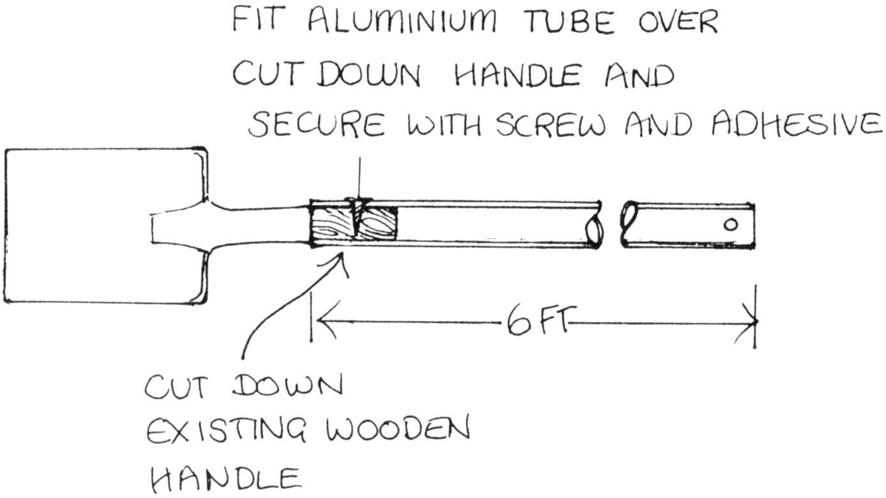

A TAD modification to extend a tool handle for a client.

Expense

Kitting yourself out with a new set of garden tools may seem like quite an expense, especially if you have not bought any tools for a while; however, doing so may enable you to do easily what before was difficult. If you value your gardening, it will be money well spent.

Some of the tools mentioned here are quite expensive; in order that gardeners have some idea of their cost, I have taken the cost of a well-known Australian 'brand name' 2-Pronged Daisy Grubber on a short handle as the standard and expressed the costs in terms of this. At the time of writing, the cost of the Daisy Grubber (the symbol  will be used from now on) was $10 at a large hardware store; thus a tool with a cost of 2× 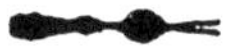 will cost $20, a tool that is 3×  will cost $30, and so forth. If the cost of the Daisy Grubber increases, then it is likely that the cost of the other tools will increase in the same proportion. Thus, if the price of the Daisy Grubber has jumped up to $11, then a tool with a cost of 2× 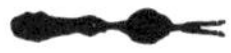 will have increased to $22, while one which costs 7× 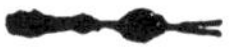 will have a price increase from $70 to $77. Tool prices are only approximate.

Try before you buy

Always try out a new tool before buying it. If you cannot actually try it in the garden, then at least hold it and simulate the action used when working with it. If you feel some strain on simply trying a tool out in the shop, then it will not be comfortable to use in the garden.

Working Positions

Working from a standing position

If, for whatever reason, you are unable to bend your back, your best option may be to work from an standing position using a tool with a long handle. It is still difficult not to bend your back when standing if you are holding the tool before you, facing the bed you are working in. By standing side-on to a garden bed, with the tool held out at your side, it is possible to work the tool through the soil by stepping from side to side. In some situations, for example, cultivating an empty garden bed, it is possible to use a tool by dragging it behind you.

Remember to check with a health professional before altering your gardening posture. Bending in the garden may be important in exercising your back; however, if you feel that it is taking the *pleasure* out of gardening, then it is probably better to alter your way of gardening and to introduce some other, more controlled form of back exercise.

There are quite a number of conventional long-handled tools available through mainstream retailers, including hoes, rakes, and cultivators. However, some may be too large, some may be too heavy, and the handles may be too short for taller individuals.

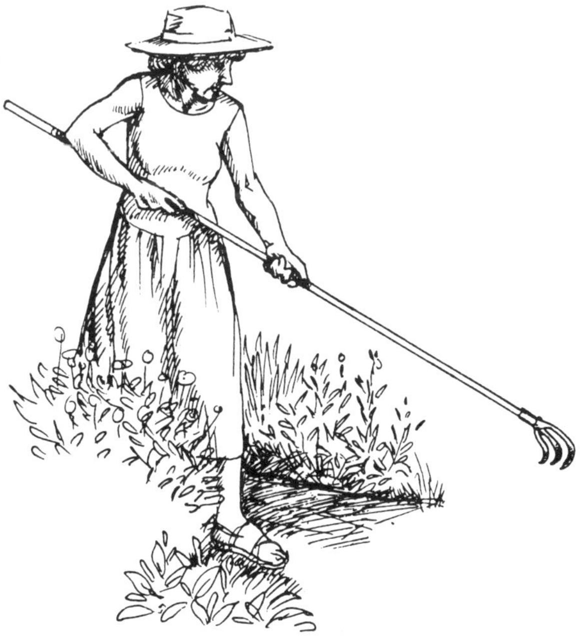

Working side-on in a standing position to avoid bending the back.

A very useful range of tools is made by the German company Wolf Tools. Their Multi-Change range features small, detachable tool-heads which snap easily and firmly into handles of varying lengths. The handle lengths range from 30 cm (1′) through to 170 cm (5′ 7″) with a number of lengths in between. Some handle lengths are available in wood or in lightweight aluminium. The 84 cm length has a T-handle, and an auxiliary D-handle can be attached to handles of any length; the T- and D-handles are useful for gardeners who work best using both hands to guide a tool. The 140 cm, 150 cm and 170 cm handles are the lengths suitable for gardening while standing. The tool-heads include a number of small hoes, cultivators and weeders, a trowel, a flower fork, a seed sower and lawn edger, and some very useful small rakes, to mention but a few. These tools are sturdy and well made and are used extensively in horticultural therapy gardens. (See photos 23 and 24.)

Wolf Tools are imported, but alas, there are no Australian-made equivalents at present. However, these tools are not fiercely expensive, and since they are very robust (the tool-heads come with a 5 year guarantee), they are value for money. Because the handle lengths can be changed to suit the task and the gardener, the system is very flexible, which can be extremely useful when there is more than one gardener in the house. Local retailers may not have a full range in stock, but are usually happy to order in pieces you want. The retailers should have a catalogue of the full range if you are unsure of what you are after. The tools are also available through the main distributors, who are listed in the back of the book.

Cost: Most Tool-heads—1.5 ×
Most Handles—1.5 ×

Working from a sitting position

Some gardeners find that working from a sitting position is a comfortable option, and there are many able-bodied older gardeners who prefer to work this way. If tools with handles of the correct length are used, then bending is reduced; for those who tire easily or have difficulties working and standing at the same time, sitting down while gardening may make the activity a straightforward and pleasant affair, where otherwise it would be an arduous, if not impossible, chore.

There are several factors to consider when choosing a working seat for the garden. Firstly, it is important that the seat is comfortable for an extended period; secondly, the seat should be small enough and light enough to be moved around the garden easily; finally, it should be quite stable so that the safety of the gardener is not jeopardised. Aspects of comfort include the height of the seat, the presence or absence of a backrest or armrests, and the material from which the chair is made. The height of the seat above the ground at which the gardener is comfortable will determine the length of the handle of the tools used to work the garden, and so *the seating is the first thing that should be selected.* If you do not have a suitable seat at home already, contemplate purchasing one of the small seats described a little later in this chapter.

It is all too easy to overreach or twist ourselves into awkward positions when working from a fixed position, so it is essential that the tools used in this position are the correct length. Conventional hoes, cultivators and rakes can have their handles shortened; the gardener may benefit from reducing the size of the tool-head as well. Wolf Tools include handles of an intermediate length (78 cm and 100 cm) in their interchangeable Multi-Change range and these are a good length for many people. There are also some tools of suitable lengths available through rehabilitation suppliers.

Gardeners with little strength in their arms often find it easier to use tools with both their hands; an additional handle fixed at right angles to the shaft of the tool can provide a better grip and far more control over a tool and may suit some older gardeners. There are a number of such auxiliary handles available, some of which are described in this chapter.

It can be a great temptation to reach 'just that little bit further' when anchored to one spot. This can lead to gardeners stretching and straining things, getting themselves into all manner of strange and contorted positions or even overbalancing, all of which can have very unpleasant consequences. It is important that we be aware of this when working; we should keep an upright posture, and make sure that we attempt to garden only those areas that can be easily reached from the spot we are sitting in.

Once again, if you are thinking of changing your working position in the garden, consult a health professional; if these changes alter the amount or the type of exercise you will receive in your daily activities, this may need to be compensated for.

Working from a kneeling position

Some older gardeners find it comfortable to work from a kneeling position, and many of these gardeners use a kneeling frame when doing so. A kneeling frame provides a firm, padded surface at ground level that is easy on the knees; handles allow the gardener to get up and down easily without bending the back.

Small handtools are suitable for using from a kneeling frame. There are a number of conventional handtools available, or the Wolf Multi-Change tool-heads can be used with the 30 cm (1′) handle.

Again, gardeners working from the fixed position of a kneeling frame may be tempted to overreach or to twist themselves into awkward—and dangerous—positions. Be sure to check with your doctor, physiotherapist or occupational therapist if contemplating a major change in your gardening ways.

The Right Tools

Tool preference is a highly individual thing, and despite the title of this section, there are no absolute rights or wrongs, there are only good choices and bad choices, according to the needs and likings of each gardener. Having examined the way in which we garden and determined which working position suits each of us best, the next step is to select tools that will serve us best in that position. Often one tool performs a number of tasks quite adequately, but sometimes a tool that has been designed for a particular task will make that task very much simpler. What follows is a list of a number of common gardening activities and a selection of garden tools designed to cope with them.

Weeding

Weeding can be the gardener's bane. There are few of us who actually enjoy doing it, though occasionally one might find oneself in a state of mind where the action is therapeutic. Usually, it is an utter chore, and one which must be done with irritating regularity. I hope in the next chapter to convince you of the wisdom of mulching your garden; this will cut down the weeding to practically nothing if done properly. Even so, there will be some need to weed occasionally; a crop of weeds is usually the first sign that the mulch in that area has composted into the soil and needs a top-up. It is usually only the most diligent and organised gardener who manages to keep ahead of such happenings, and weeding remains a necessity for most.

Most of us must weed amongst established plants, where each weed must be removed individually. A certain amount of precision is called for; the following tools may be of use:

Multi-change tools. There is a number of tool-heads that are designed for weeding in the Wolf range: Weeding fork, push-pull weeder, cultiweeder and others. Combine these with a handle of the correct length for your needs. (See photo 23.)

Trigger-operated weeder. The Baronet Long Reach Weeder is made by a UK company and imported here by rehabilitation suppliers. It is a little like a long-handled apple corer operated by a trigger action. The business end of the tool is inserted into the ground to encircle the offending weed. When the trigger is pulled, the 'thumb' of the gadget grips the weed which can then be lifted out. This last action requires that the gardener have a certain amount of strength in their hand. The tool is 864 mm (34″) long; at my height of 157 cm (5′ 2″), I find it a good length, but taller gardeners will have to stoop a little when using it. It is comfortable to use while sitting down, but is unsuitable for hard, unworked soils. Available from rehabilitation suppliers. (See photo 28.)

Cost: 13× [redacted] +22% sales tax

Foot-pedal lawn weeders. There are two locally made weeders available that are operated by a foot-pedal. Both tools will remove weeds from garden beds as well as lawns, but since they are operated by a foot-pedal, it usually means trampling all over the garden bed to use them. A reasonable amount of balance is needed to use either of them.

The mainstream tool company Cyclone make a long-handled lawn weeder that is specifically designed for broadleafed weeds, such as dandelions, that have a nice, definite root system—it is not meant for fine weeds or weeds with running root systems, such as couch and kikuyu. It is 111 cm (44″) from top to toe, and at 1.5 kg (3 lb 5 oz), weighs about the same as a garden spade. (See photo 26—tool nearest window.)

Cost: 4×

The small Western Australian Company Tanyana manufacture a very simple foot-pedal weeder. It consists of a wooden handle with aluminium prongs at the base. The prongs are inserted into the weed by pushing with the foot on the top end of the foot-pedal; the sprung lever is then depressed with the foot and the weeds are lifted clear of the ground. It retains quite a clump of soil along with the weed roots, and is best suited to lighter soils. The weeder is 111 cm long and weighs 1.7 kg (3 lb 12 oz). (See photos 29 and 30.)

Cost: 5× plus postage

Harpoon weeder. Made by Wolf Tools, this weeder comes on a 75 cm (2′ 6″) handle with a T-grip. It is inserted in the ground next to the roots of the weed, then rotated to remove the invader. It is a little ripper—literally, making short work of weeds with a discreet root system, such as dandelions, thistles, bitter cress, petty spurge and even the dread oxalis. Weeds come out with a neat plug of soil attached to the roots. (See photo 25.)

The handle length means taller gardeners will have to stoop to use it from a standing position, but it is a good length to use while sitting.

Cost: 2.5×

Miscellaneous. There is a number of hoes and cultivators that are made by the mainstream tool companies; many of these are useful for weeding and are discussed in the next section.

Cultivating—(Digging and hoeing)

Cultivation can be counter-productive. In the next chapter I have discussed this in some depth in the section on soils; my hope is that I can win you over to 'no-dig' gardening techniques. Each time you cultivate your soil, you break up whatever soil structure has been formed by the action of soil-dwelling organisms on the minerals and the organic matter contained in the soil. One of the most important effects of these soil-dwellers is the stabilisation of the relatively large soil spaces that hold the air. Air in the soil is essential for plants to carry out many different functions, and without it, plants can literally suffocate. Cultivation improves aeration, but only for a very short period of time. Without the 'glue' of secretions from these organisms (worms, fungi, bacteria) and from plant roots, the air spaces created by turning over the soil will soon collapse. Unless organic matter is regularly added to the soil *and* the resultant brew left to 'cook', the only way to 'open up' the soil is to cultivate it—either by turning it over with a fork or spade, or by using a hoe or cultivator. If you are a traditionalist, you will probably continue turning over the soil for your annual plantings, be they vegetables or spring flowers. Here are some tools that may make this task a little easier:

Digging

Small spades and forks. Hardware stores and garden centres often stock small spades and forks. They are sold under several appellations—'Light Border', 'Ladies'', 'Campers'', 'Auto'—and may come with a T- or a D- handle; all will have relatively short handles which may require lengthening to allow easy use.

There is also an important range of very light, very elegant long-handled tools with small, stainless steel work-heads with lightweight aluminium handles. Made by the UK company Bulldog, the range includes a small fork, a rake and a Dutch hoe (See photo 27). They are available through the Australian head office of Wolf Tools.

Cost: 6×

Stainless steel tools. Tools made from stainless steel are lighter and soils will not stick to them to the same extent as it will to tools made of other materials. Because of this, they will take fewer 'passes' to move a given amount of soil, and be that bit lighter to lift when emptied, as they shed their load more efficiently.

Foot-operated autospade. Wolf Tools make a foot-operated 'Terrex Autospade' which allows the gardener to dig in an upright position without lifting either the tool or the soil. It is easy to use once you adjust to the rather different action that is needed to operate it. Firstly, the spade is lowered into the soil; when the foot-pedal is depressed, the spring-loaded lever which is attached to the pedal lifts the blade out of the soil, along with its load. The blade is then emptied of its load by rotating the handles through 120 degrees, and the whole process repeated. The arms do most of the work and bending is unnecessary. The tool is slightly heavier than a conventional spade but need not be lifted out of the ground once it is in use. (See photos 37 and 38.)

Cost: 13×

The 'ergonomic' tool range. These tools are somewhat of a departure from the conventional tool design. With their S-bend handles, the Ergonomic tools have been designed to allow their use in an improved posture, where the user's back is less bent, and the load is more evenly distributed across the body. Their enterprising young designer, Peter Fegan, is a former landscaper. Years of shifting topsoil and sand made him aware of the shortcomings of conventional shovels, and after a bit of trial and error, he came up with his first innovative design, the Ergonomic Shovel (see photo 35). He had the design tested by physiotherapists and chiropractors, who pronounced it sound. One engineer involved in the testing commented:

> It is a source of amazement that such a simple, economical modification which has effects of such a magnitude has not been incorporated before now.

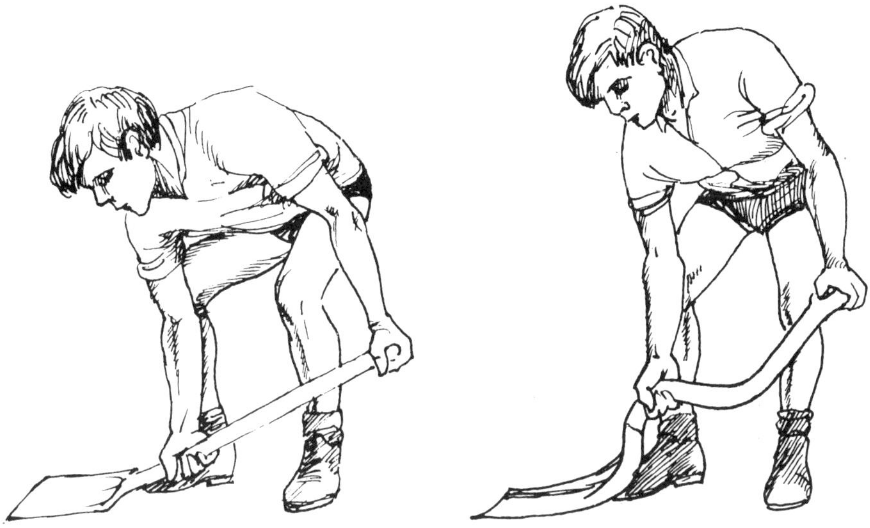

The working posture for the 'Ergonomic Shovel'.

The Ergonomic range now includes several styles of spades, shovels and a fork, each with a bend in the shaft appropriate to the action needed to use it (see photo 36). I find it makes a great difference to the work involved. As someone without a huge amount of physical strength, I find it lessens the strain enormously. I wouldn't be without mine!

Cost: 3× plus postage

Hoes and cultivators

Hoes and cultivators are used for working soil that is maintained in a fine tilth for growing vegetables and other annual crops. They are used for making the soil more penetrable to air and water, for weeding, and for sundry purposes such as making seed drills and mounding up the soil. They are sometimes used for scarifying, that is, scraping off the water-resistant crust that forms on some soils, or for removing mosses and liverworts. Some gardeners use them for weeding garden beds, though there is always the danger of damaging the roots of your garden plants when doing this; however, it is possible to avoid injuring your planting when weeding with a hoe if due caution and care are observed.

Conventional tools. Conventional tool manufacturers make a range of different hoes and cultivators of traditional design, each of which is intended for a slightly different purpose. The use to which they will eventually be put depends less on their design than on how the gardener sees fit to use them; some gardeners find them extremely helpful, others find them of no use at all.

Multi-change tools. The Wolf Multi-Change tool-heads include many of the traditional hoes and cultivators plus a number of more recently developed designs. (See photo 23.)

'Aussie Hoe'. This is a 'new improved model' of a traditional tri-sided chipping hoe. Its improvement consists of, firstly, a serrated edge which can cut through weed growth, and secondly, an indentation at one apex, which effectively creates two prongs. (See photo 26.) These prongs enable the tool to be used as a weeder as well as a hoe and its narrow apex enables the gardener to work up close to garden plants. Its designer is an award winning Australian inventor-manufacturer who usually designs large farm machinery, but occasionally turns his hand to inventing things 'that will make people's lives a bit easier'. It comes on a broom-length wooden handle and is an inexpensive and versatile tool.

Cost: 1.5×

Auxiliary handles and other add-ons

Some gardeners find it useful to have an additional grip to direct their garden tools when weeding, hoeing and so forth. When used to provide a second handle in this way, the handles also help to spread the load more evenly across the body. There are three styles of these 'add-on' handles available. Choose from the Wolf 'Auxiliary D-Handle', the 'Attach-A-Handle' or the 'Pistol-Grip Handle'. These last two are available from rehabilitation suppliers. (See photos 31–33.)

The Pistol-Grip Handle can also be used with small hand tools so that the tools can be used by gardeners with weak wrists or a poor grip. The handles are angled so that the tools can be grasped in a more ergonomically sound way causing less strain for the gardener. A range of hand tools with these angled handles is also available; these are described in a later section (Aids for Gardeners with Special Needs).

The Attach-A-Handle can also be used as a small extender if a tool handle is a little too short. This is more useful than it might sound. Even though I am small, I often find tools are just that bit shorter than is comfortable and these small handles have proved very handy as instant extenders.

Cost: D-Handle— 2×
Attach-A-Handle— 2×
Pistol-Grip Handle— 3×

Universal Back Saver. The Universal Back Saver is an attachment that allows tools such as spades and shovels to be used with a levering action from a standing position. This reduces the work required by the back and relocates the effort needed to the arms and upper body. Gardeners with strong arms may find this add-on useful in the garden;

others will find it of more use on the vacuum cleaner. The medium duty model is recommended for the home gardener. (See photo 34.)

Cost: 3× +postage

Building up handle grips. Some gardeners, especially those with arthritis in their hands, may work more comfortably with the handles of their tools built up a little to make them wider. Rehabilitation suppliers sell various materials, including foam tubing and a mouldable, clay-like substance, which can be used to enlarge tool handles, making them easier to grip.

Kneeling frames

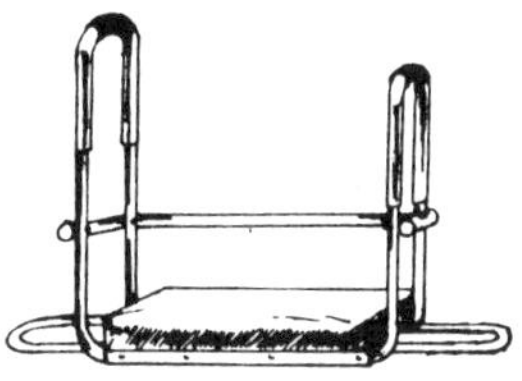

Asymmetrical kneeler.

Many older gardeners find it comfortable to use a kneeling frame in the garden. Many hardware stores stock a basic kneeling frame or kneeler, with a light polystyrene foam pad for kneeling and a tubular aluminium frame with a hooked handle.

Cost: 3×

A more substantial kneeler is available through the R. E. Ross Centre at Caulfield General Hospital in Melbourne. Their standard kneeling frame features an upholstered kneeling pad and has strong handles that loop all the way over; this will be of benefit to gardeners who must lean heavily on the handles to get up and down. The Ross Centre also make an asymmetrical kneeling frame for people who have the use of only one arm.

Cost: Standard— 4.5× +postage
Asymmetrical— 8× +postage

Rehabilitation suppliers stock two different kneeling frames which can be turned upside-down and used as a seat. The 'Kneel N Sit' has a polystyrene kneeling pad which is used as a cushion when the frame is used as a seat. It has small handles to assist with getting up and down in either position. The 'Easi Kneeler' has more substantial handles to aid the gardener when getting on or off the frame when used as either a seat or a kneeler, and has a soft padded cushion. (See photos 19–21.) It is, however, a little heavier than the Kneel N Sit.

Cost: Kneel N Sit— 8.5× +22% sales tax
Easi Kneeler— 14× +22% sales tax

Seats

The first gardener I ever knew to weed sitting down was a retired farmer who had moved from a citrus farm in Mildura to a Melbourne suburb. She brought with her a one-legged disc seat from an old horse-drawn plough. On this agrarian antique she sits and tends her garden, with the leg of the disc seat firmly anchored in the ground. When she has finished, this septuagenarian gardener simply lifts the seat out of the ground and moves it on to the next spot.

While few of us will have such picturesque structures to sit upon whilst working, it is nevertheless possible to buy suitable small, light but stable seats. The Kneel N Sit and the Easi Kneeler kneeling frames described above are versatile pieces of equipment that convert to seats just by turning them upside-down. The 'Met-A-Lite Garden Stool' is a small gardening work seat designed for people who have difficulty getting up and down. It is made by a small NSW manufacturing company. Like a kneeling frame, it has tubular handles and a padded vinyl seat 30 cm (1′) off the ground; it does not have a back rest.

Cost: Met-A-Lite Garden Stool—8.5× +postage

Small portable 'Golfers' seats can be useful if you use one that is solid and stable. If you need a back rest, or if stability is a problem for you, a lightweight outdoors seat may serve you well, but avoid fold-up seats. Whatever you sit on, make sure that it is a comfortable height for you to work from.

Lugging and carting

There is often much carting and lugging about to be done in the garden; weeds, prunings, lawn clippings must be removed, while mulch, fertiliser and sometimes water must be delivered. It is important that this carrying be done safely, in a way that causes no damage to the gardener. Serious injury can, and frequently does, result from carrying things badly in the garden. Indeed, during our most recent drought, there was an epidemic of back complaints caused by carting buckets of water out to the garden during the water restrictions.

There are two aspects of moving things around in the garden that we need to attend to. The first of these is our lifting and carrying technique; these I will cover a little later in the chapter. The second of these aspects is the equipment that we use to assist us. I have listed some helpful implements below.

Garden grippers. Garden grippers are devices which allow the gardener to pick up the leaves, lawn clippings and so forth without bending. They are comprised of two paddle-like end plates that scoop up and carry the load, and two handles which open and close the end plates with a scissor action. The handles are long enough—around 80 cm (32″)—to eliminate most of the bending. There are two styles of garden grippers available in Australia. The first is the locally designed and produced 'Garden Gillie' (See photo 44). Its designer-manufacturer made the first one for his wife when she 'slipped a disc' almost twenty years ago. Requests from family and friends finally convinced him to produce them commercially. The second is an imported gripper available from rehabilitation suppliers; this differs from the local version in having angled handgrips at the top to allow comfortable gripping.

Cost: Local— 4.5×
Imported—6× +22% Sales Tax

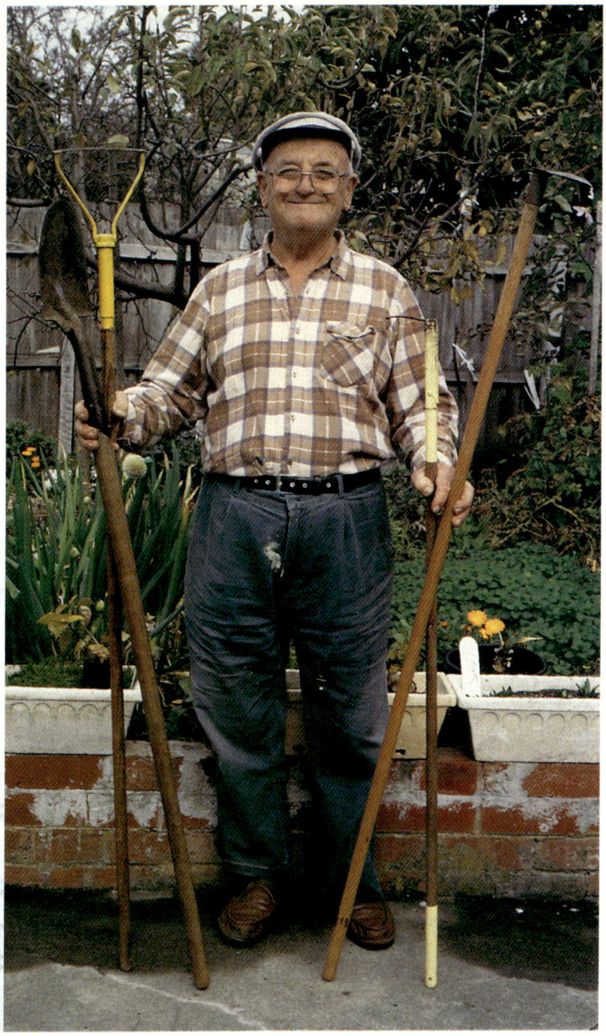

13

Steve Stephenson *with gardening tools he made himself*

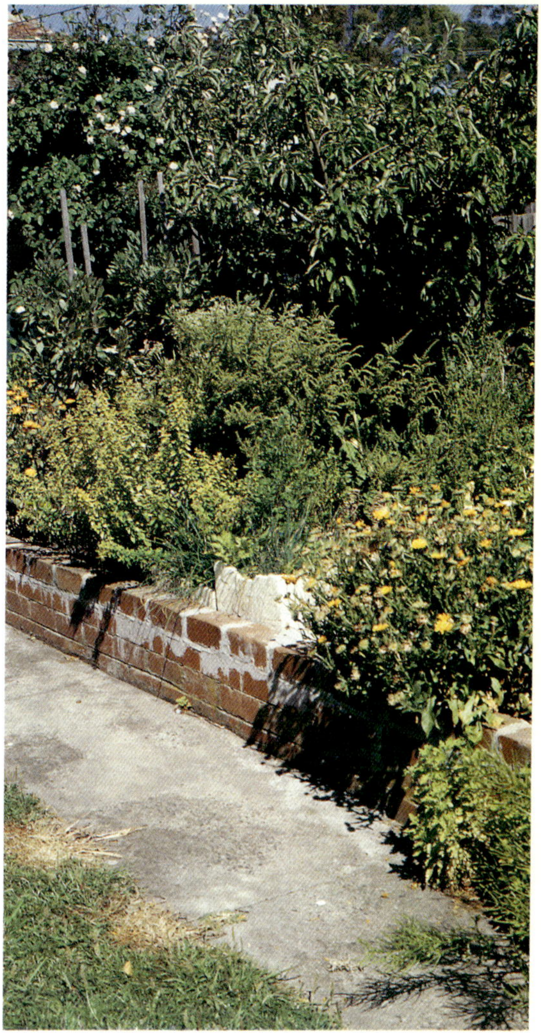

14

Steve Stephenson's raised vegetable garden

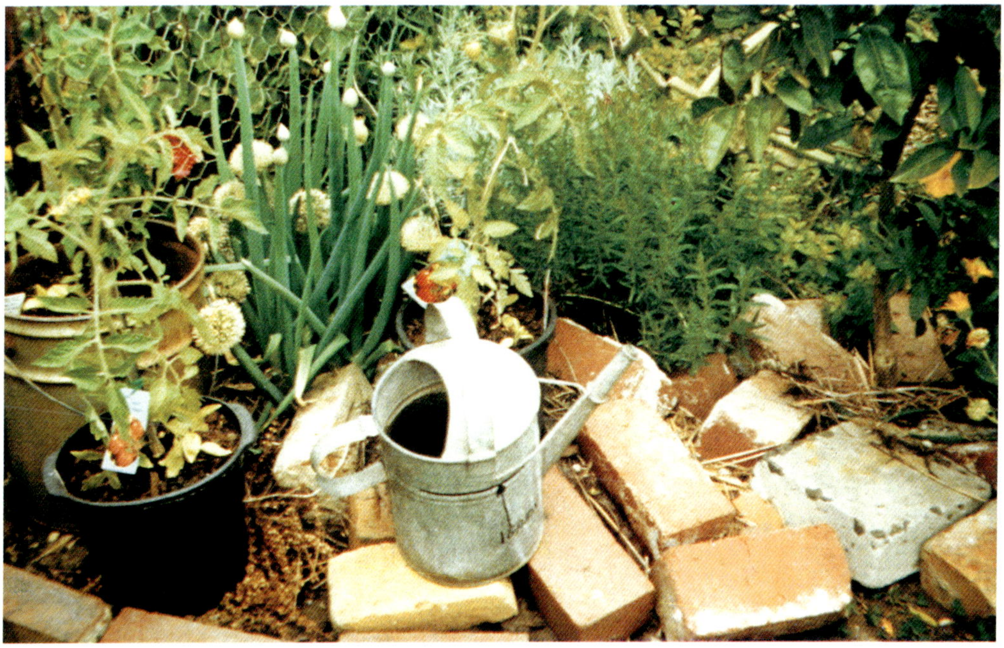

Brick-mulched herbs and fruit tree in the Stephenson garden

15

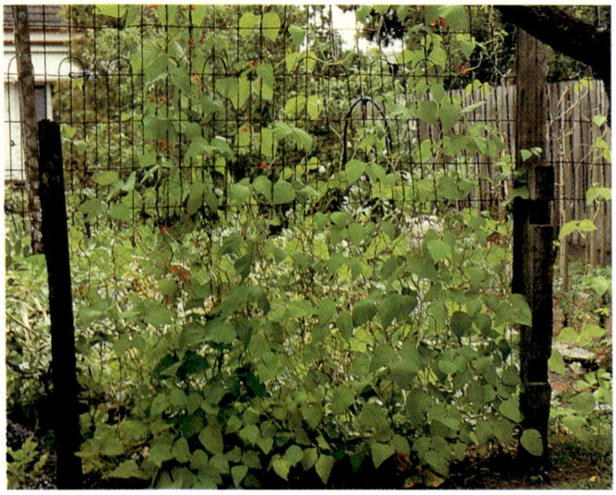

Mary Watson's vegetable garden in early summer 16

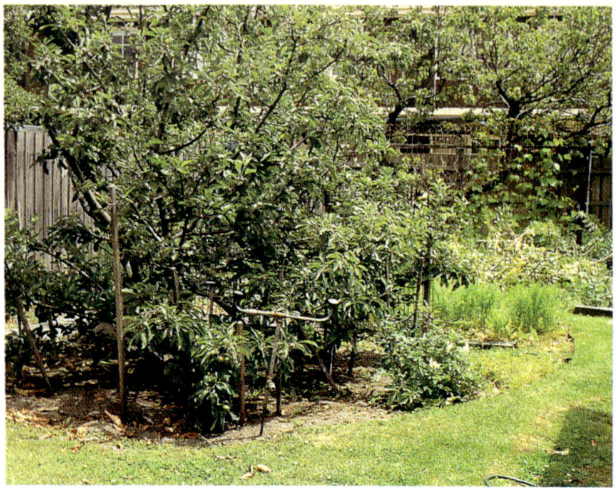

A view of the apple trees in the back garden 17

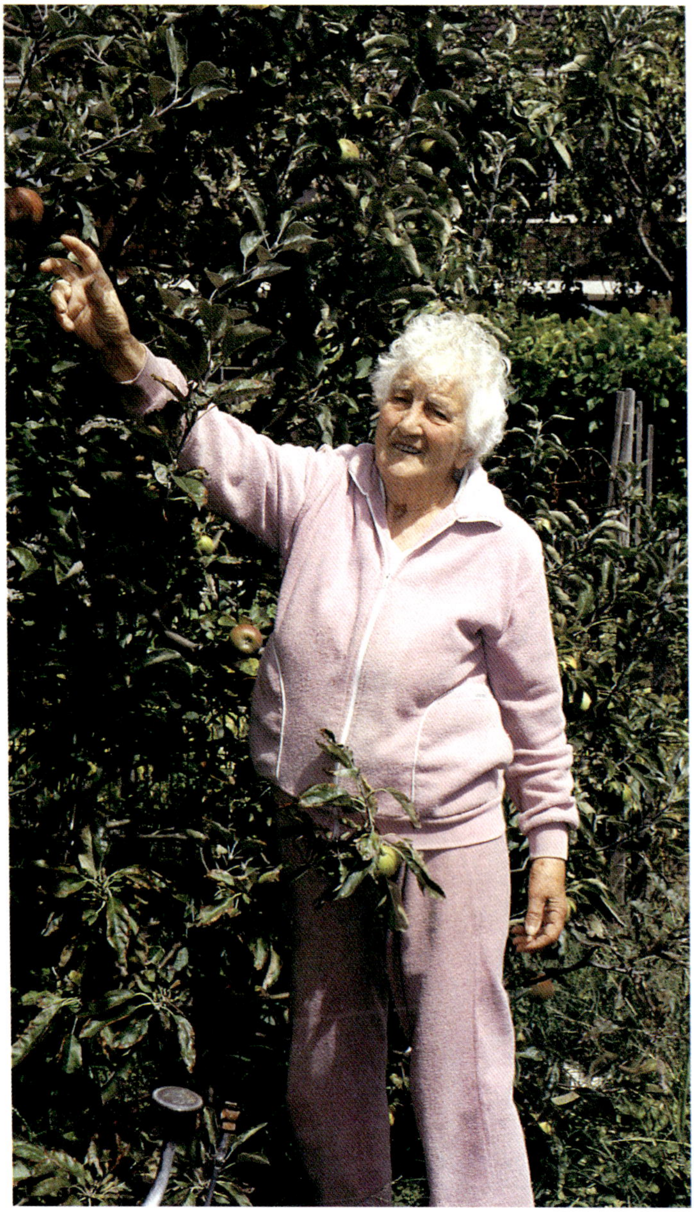

Mary Watson *and one of her multiple-grafted apple trees* 18

Rakes. Small leaf rakes can be used for a multitude of tasks around the garden, and can cut out a lot of bending—it is often just a matter of thinking ahead and having the tool with you when you need it. Plastic leaf rakes can be cut down to the desired size using a fine-toothed hack saw. The Wolf Multi-Change tools include an excellent small garden sweep; this sweep is one of my most treasured tools, I find it especially useful for spreading compost and mulch around my plants (see photo 47). Another useful small rake is the Bulldog stainless steel tool mentioned earlier.

Wheeled carts. Wheelbarrows are the gardener's usual choice of wheeled cart, but this is an area where a little lateral thinking may turn up a better alternative. Laundry trolleys are a light and inexpensive way of transporting tools, fertiliser and mulch around the garden, and the goods can be reached without bending. Wire shopping jeeps are also useful for the same reasons (I mean the wire jeeps one *buys*, not supermarket trolleys), and even cane or vinyl shopping jeeps can be useful with a small tray or box placed on top to carry things.

Two-wheeled wheelbarrows are much easier to use than conventional barrows with only one wheel. The 'Daytek' twin-wheeled cart has pneumatic tyres; it is pulled rather than pushed, which means that more of your energy goes into moving the barrow forward than is the case with push-along barrows; consequently, less energy is expended moving a given load in a two wheeler than in its one-wheeled equivalent. The handle of the twin-wheeled barrow is at waist height so that much bending is avoided; it is available at larger hardware stores. (See photo 43.)

Cost: 8.5×

The 'Ascender Lift Barrows' are a range of wheelbarrows with a tray that can be lowered onto the ground for loading and unloading. The tray is lifted on and off the wheels using a levering action on the handles; this is simply done by walking along the barrow while holding one handle. The barrows come in three different sizes; the smallest (the 'Minor') has a load capacity of 100 kg (220 lb 7 oz) and should be large enough for most home gardeners. The next two sizes up (the 'Major' and the 'Magnum') have load capacities of 150 kg (330 lb 10½ oz) and 250 kg (551 lb 1½ oz) respectively. Specify 'Twin' when ordering, as the two smaller sizes are also available with a single wheel. All have large pneumatic tyres and can be obtained from their NSW manufacturer.

Cost: Minor Twin— 29× +postage
Major Twin— 32× +postage
Magnum Twin—41× +postage

Pruning

There are three types of pruning tools that may be of interest to older gardeners. They are the 'cut and hold' secateurs, ratchet secateurs, and the long-handled pruning saws and loppers.

Cut and hold secateurs. Cut and hold secateurs are made by several companies including Wolf Tools and Kamaki. They range from conventional hand-held anvil secateurs (see photo 39) to long-handled trigger-operated pruners. (See photos 40 and 41.) These pruners can be particularly useful on two counts. Firstly, they allow the gardener to work one-handed so that flowers and fruit can be cut and picked in the same operation while prunings can be recovered and disposed of without the need to bend. Secondly, the long-handled pruners allow the gardener to extend their reach into the garden; they are quite lightweight and can be particularly helpful if the gardener is working from a fixed position (sitting or kneeling). This also means that it is unnecessary to risk life and limb perching on ladders while picking fruit, cleaning out climbers and all those other jobs that are normally out of reach from the ground. These implements are not heavy-duty and can only be used for lighter pruning.

Cost: Wolf and hand-held 'Cut-and-Hold' secateurs—5.5 ×
Kamaki trigger-operated 'Cut-and-Hold' secateurs:
Medium Reach (64 cm or 2′ 1″)—7 ×
Long Reach (150 cm or 5′)—9.5 ×

Ratchet secateurs. Ratchet secateurs allow the gardener to cut using little effort—repeated small actions from the gardener will eventually cut through quite thick branches. The 'Easy-Grip Secateurs' will cut through up to 19 mm (0.75″). These well-made English pruners are available through the large rehabilitation suppliers; they are strong and well-made, but are rather more expensive than the ratchet pruners that occasionally appear on the supermarket shelves.

Cost: Easy-Grip Secateurs—3.5 × + 22% Sales Tax

Heavy-duty, long-handled pruners. A number of mainstream tool companies make heavy-duty long-handled pruners. These include long-handled scissor-action loppers and high-reach tools on the end of poles. Both pulley-operated pruners for lighter pruning (up to 3 cm or 1 inch, depending on the quality of the tool) and pruning saws for the heavier pruning are available. An attachment for picking fruit is available with the Wolf Multi-Change range. The poles are usually sold separately and the gardener sometimes has the choice of a wooden pole or a lightweight, adjustable telescopic handle. All these pruners need both hands to operate them; a fair degree of physical strength is also required to lift and steady them when in use.

Watering equipment

Watering the garden by hand is a task that some gardeners find highly therapeutic, while others find it tedious in the extreme. If you fall into the latter category, then you probably will have taken steps to reduce the amount of watering you need to do. Hopefully you will have mulched and introduced a watering system; if not, Chapters 4 and 5 will be of interest to you. If, on the other hand, you enjoy getting out there and pointing the hose at your plants, there is something that you should know.

Water is like a drug of addiction to plants—the more you give them, the more they need. Plants that are given frequent waterings develop only shallow root systems; they are then unable to reach deeper-lying water, and so are dependent on regular waterings. In contrast, plants which are watered deeply but infrequently will develop deep roots to seek out the lower-lying moisture. So giving your plants a brief squirt at the end of a long hot day may refresh *you*, but ultimately it will do little for your garden; try to curb your zeal and restrict your daily watering to pots and other containers which do need watering frequently. If you redirect your energies into mulching your garden, you will have happier plants *and* a lower water bill. See Chapter 4 for a full discussion on the hows and whys of mulching.

Container-grown plants will need frequent watering. How often will depend on the size of the container, the water-retaining properties of the growing medium, the weather conditions, and the individual needs of the plants. Chapter 6 contains further information on growing plants in pots. It is possible to install a watering system to deal with plants in containers (see Chapter 5), and if you have a number of pots it will be well worth your while. Modern watering systems made of PVC are very flexible. If you decide to move your plants around, the watering outlets can be easily moved too, simply by inserting the dripper or the sprayer in the new spot, and plugging the hole left behind. If you have only a few plants growing in pots, or if you enjoy watering each plant individually, make sure that you are doing it in a way that is easy on your back (see 'Good Habits' below).

Hand-held hoses are the easiest and most efficient way to water your plants by hand. Various attachments such as trigger-operated soft spray 'guns' are available to regulate the flow of water from the hose, making it gentle enough for watering container-grown plants. Long-handled guns make it possible to water hanging baskets and out-of-reach containers without strain.

These guns stop the waterflow at the nozzle when the triggers are not depressed. This can be very convenient, but *the water should always be turned off at the tap* when you have finished watering. The seals on these devices can give under prolonged pressure, causing havoc when they do. My sister once emptied out the entire contents of a water tank this way one summer—it was the sole water supply for the household, and they had to buy in water for the rest of the season. With water a scarce resource for much of our continent, and a costly one for the rest, wasting water is something we none of us can afford to do.

Hose holders. Hose holders may also be useful for those who find it difficult to manage a hose. These consist of a spiked metal rod of around 80 cm (2′ 7½″) that can be pushed into the ground; the hose nozzle is held near the top of the rod by either a clamp or a split ring frame which can then be adjusted to direct the spray. They are inexpensive and may be more useful than sprinklers in some situations.

Cost: 2×  + postage

Always leave your hose wound up and out of the way when not in use. A hose left lying across a path or in the lawn is quite easily overlooked and can cause a gardener to come quite a cropper (no pun intended). There are many hose reels on the market, ranging from a simple arc reel that is mounted on the wall (and which costs only a few dollars) to an auto-rewind reel which costs considerably more!

If you water using a bucket or a watering can, you will be aware of just how heavy water is. It is vital that you carry no more than is comfortable for you, that your posture is good and the weight evenly distributed across your body. These issues are discussed more fully in the following section.

Aids for Gardeners with Special Needs

Working one-handed

Gardeners who must work one-handed may find this modified crutch useful for working with long-handled tools. A leather 'gutter' secures the tool to the forearm by means of velcro straps, while a handgrip at right angles to the handle makes it easier to guide the tool. Information on this adaptation can be obtained from the Independent Living Centres.

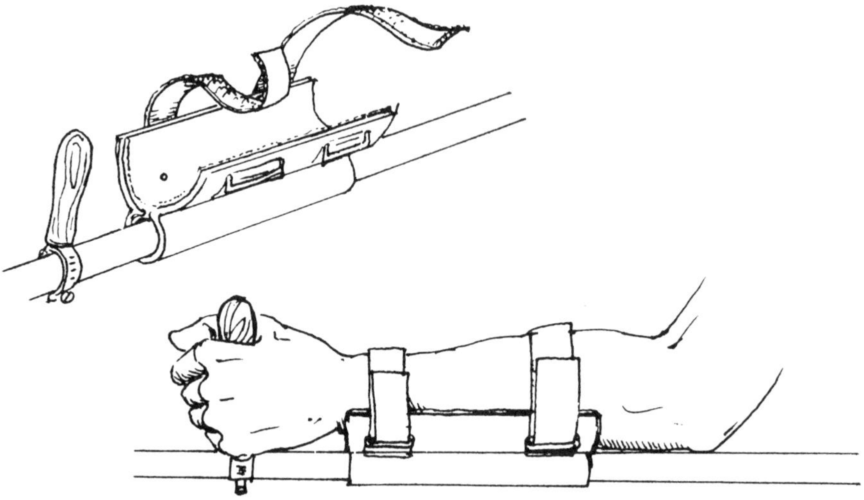

ILC adaptation to long-handled tools to allow one-handed use.

Angle-grip garden hand tools

The 'Peta Fist Grip Garden Tools' have an angled handle that allows them to be gripped in a 'fist', and are useful for gardeners with weak hands and wrists. All tools are available with a short handle (trowel, fork, cultivator, hoe, two-pronged weeder); all but the weeder are also available on a longer handle (76 cm or 2′ 6″) suitable for using while seated.

Cost: Short-handled tools—3.5× +postage
Long reach tools— 5× +postage

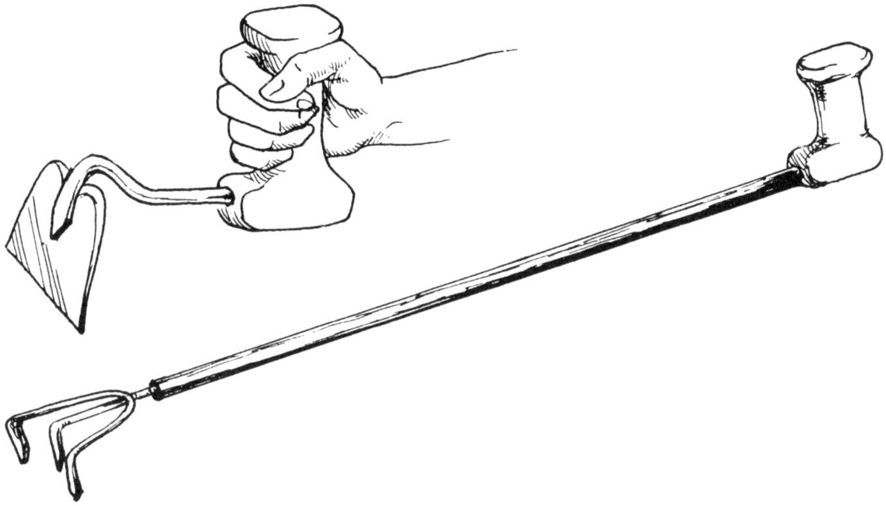

Angle-Grip hand tools: short-handled hoe; long-reach.

Mobile gardening chair

This is a garden seat with wheels, a backrest, and a tray for carrying tools. A plastic moulded seat and armrests are optional extras. The gardener can propel the chair along when seated, by pushing against the ground using their feet, or the gardener can be pushed by an assistant. The seat height is adjustable within certain limits using a wing-nut.

Good Habits

I initially called this section 'Self-Discipline', but then thought that perhaps a title like that would cause most readers to skip over it. Yet a little gentle self-discipline in the garden is often called for; how many times do we go into the garden just to do some little job (trim a shrub, pull a weed, cut a flower), and find ourselves still there three hours later, happy but a trifle weary? And how often do we find ourselves suffering from the aftermath of those happy hours, wishing that we had not worked for quite so long? I know many's the time that I have done it. Finally, I have learnt to limit the damage by planning my gardening and controlling both the time and the tasks of each gardening session. I now work with a definite, though informal, action plan.

Action plans

It is important to think about both the total time that we work in the garden, and how long we spend at each particular task. Rest breaks should be taken at regular intervals. It is important, too, that we limit the time spent on any one activity, and vary our actions in order to avoid even small doses of Repetitive Strain Injury. For example, if you start off weeding at ground level, you could follow it with pruning a little higher, then with raking up some leaves or carrying some clippings to the compost heap; this combination will exercise different parts of you in different ways. After working through it, return to weeding and repeat the whole cycle again.

Just how long you can spend on each task will depend on both your own level of fitness and the demands of the job in question. It is so easy to drift off into an almost trance-like state when gardening, loosing track of both time and the state of our bodies. If this happens to you, as I know it does to me, it is a good idea to take pen and paper and a clock out with you into the garden a few times, to try to establish just where your limits lie. Record just how long you work for, and at what, record when you start to feel sore or weary, and also how you feel afterwards. That way, you will get the measure of it, and be able to pace yourself accordingly. Set yourself reasonable limits *and stick to them*, timing yourself by the clock if necessary.

Schedule regular rest breaks throughout your gardening session. Do it properly—have a cuppa in your favourite spot, read the paper, watch the birds, or anything else that will give you pleasure. While it may seem at first that you don't get as much done in several short sessions as you would in one longer one, you will soon realise that by coming to the garden fresh each time, you work more efficiently. Furthermore, you will be able to go back and do it all again tomorrow—something which will definitely *not* be the case if you overdo things. Remember, one of the joys of retirement is that you *don't* have to squeeze all your gardening into the weekends.

If you find it irritating taking tools in and out each time, streamline the whole operation by storing your gardening equipment in a trolley or wheelbarrow; then the whole thing can just be wheeled in and out of the work area as required. As well as your tools, include buckets for debris, twine or plant ties, gardening gloves, fertiliser, and anything else you find yourself using with any regularity. I keep all my bits and pieces on a vegetable rack on wheels. By putting small amounts of fertiliser into old icecream tubs I keep the load neat, light and waterproof; my empty buckets and any occasionals such as seedlings go on the top, while my handtools, kneeling pad and other paraphernalia fit comfortably on the shelves underneath. The whole thing wheels easily around the lawn and while I still have to carry my larger tools out separately, this little trolley has considerably simplified my beginnings and endings in the garden. A gardening apron or belt-pouch with capacious pouches for hand tools is useful when a larger range of tools is not required.

Pain

Never do anything to the point of pain. Always stop the *instant* you feel the slightest twinge. Resist the urge to 'just finish this job'—pain is an indication that something is being damaged! It is all too easy to drift off when gardening and neglect to monitor the state of our bodies—try to maintain an awareness of your physical state at all times.

If you find that you have been working in the one position for some time and things are starting to ache, come out of the position slowly and gradually, then gently stretch *away* from the pain several times until it starts to ease. At one stage, I would often get caught bending over weeding for too long, and still occasionally do, I blush to confess. To combat this, I stretch upwards with my hands above my head, arching my back until the pain abates and I start to feel my muscles relaxing back into their normal state. Usually ten arches does the trick, but I have been known to get up to sixteen before recovering. Until I learnt to do this simple exercise, I would often 'seize up' and find myself unable to straighten my back, and in some degree of pain. It is, however, a *last resort*, and is nowhere near as effective as *not overdoing it in the first place*!

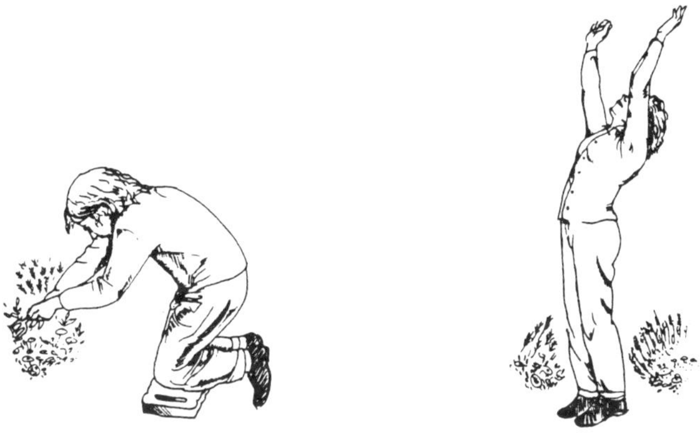

If you start to experience pain after bending over for long, stretch away from the pain, arching your back until the pain eases.

Posture

Good posture is as important in the garden as it is anywhere else. It is especially important that our basic working positions are sound, that nothing is strained or twisted before we even start. All the usual advice of 'bend at the knees, don't slump, keep your back straight' applies just as much, if not more, in the garden as in other areas of your life. Remember that joints such as knees and elbows were designed with bending rather more in mind than were backs; try always to let the other joints do the work and give your back a break wherever possible. Similarly, arm and leg muscles are able to take more strain when lifting and carrying—give them the work to do, not your back.

Lifting and carrying

Never lift anything that is too big or too heavy for you to carry. If possible, break a load up into small, manageable parts. If this is not possible, get help. Don't put your back at risk because it seems easier to attempt the job yourself rather than asking for assistance—you may be paying for your hastiness for the rest of your life! With back problems as prevalent as they are, you will probably find yourself with a circle of acquaintances needing similar help, some of them relatively young. Mutual support groups often develop amongst such individuals—I know this has happened amongst my friends—and often these groups will have acquired access to a trolley or cart that will allow the load to be moved safely.

If the load is within your limits, make sure you do the following when lifting:

Get right in close to the object you are to lift.

Always keep your back straight—if you must bend to reach the object, bend your knees, not your back. Keep your back straight *at all times* while lifting.

Put your arms under or around the object and hug it in close to you when lifting. If the object is too big or too awkward in shape for you to do this comfortably, then do not attempt the lift—find an alternative way to move it.

When carrying loads such as weeds or leaves in the garden, do so in small quantities equally divided between two buckets, carrying a bucket in each hand. Carrying a lop-sided load puts a further strain on your body—take both buckets out with you at the start of your gardening session and divide everything equally between them as you go. Keep an eye on how full they are, and empty them before they get too heavy.

If watering by hand, which is sometimes necessary when water is restricted, use two buckets for this, and don't overfill them—carry only as much as you can manage easily. It will do neither yourself nor your plants any good if you damage your back. If you use a watering can, leave it at the garden bed and carry the water in the two buckets to the watering can.

Using a conventional wheelbarrow

When using a conventional one-wheeled barrow, it is easy to fall into bad habits. We are seldom educated on how to use our bodies to avoid strain during such activities, but there is a right and a wrong way to wheel a barrow, and using the right way can make all the difference to the outcome of an afternoon's gardening. The right way is to:

Stand in close to the barrow, right between the handles.

Bend your knees until your hands can grip the handles.

Stand up by straightening your legs. Keep your back straight—let your arms and legs do the work rather than your back.

Use your arms to lift the barrow ready for wheeling.

Wheel the barrow, keeping your body within the handles. *Your thumbs should remain in close to your side at all times*—this way, your back should remain straight throughout the entire proceedings.

Remember never to overload the barrow. You will ultimately save yourself time and much fatigue by taking smaller loads.

Pre-gardening warm-up exercises

As with any form of physical exercise, it is easier to strain a cold muscle than a warm one when gardening. If you know that you are going to be working a particular group of muscles hard or you have any problems with joint mobility or some other medical problem, it is a good idea to do some warm-up exercises before you start; this is especially true in cold weather. If you are already under medical supervision for anything involving the back, muscles, joints, or your overall health (such as high blood pressure or a heart complaint), ask your doctor or physiotherapist for some suitable exercises. If you have no particular health problems, the following set of exercises will help you warm up, while the last two will also help strengthen some often neglected muscles that we should be using when gardening.

A. SHOULDER ROLLS

Rotate both shoulders together, first forwards, then backwards. Repeat 5 times in each direction.

B. HIGH STEP MARCHING

March up and down on the spot, raising your knees up high as you step, and swinging your arms across your chest. Repeat 5 times.

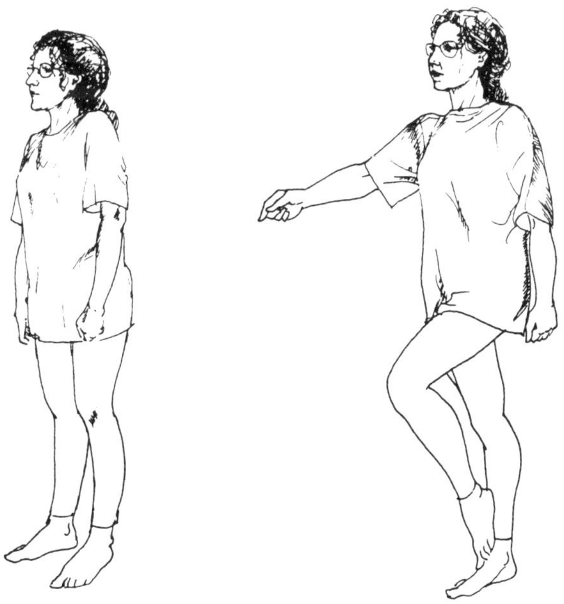

Warm-up exercises:
A—Shoulder rolls
B—High step marching

C. SINGLE KNEE CURLS

Lie flat on your back. Curl both knees up towards chest, hold for 5 seconds, then release. Repeat 5 times.

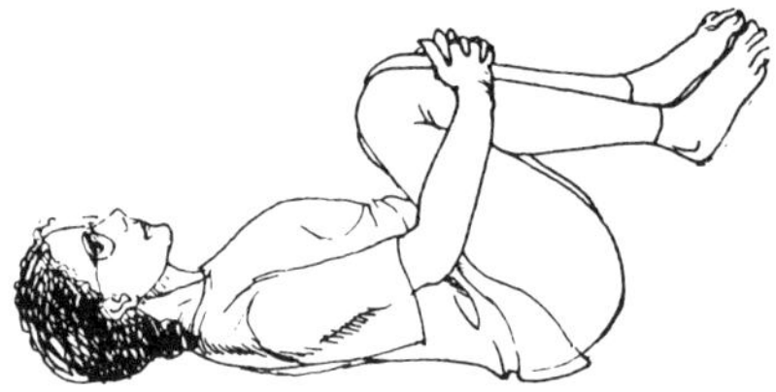

C—Single knee curls

D. WALL SQUATS

Lean back against the wall with feet a little way out from the wall; lower the body by bending the knees, but go no lower than is comfortable. Hold for 10 seconds, then straighten the knees. Repeat 5 times.

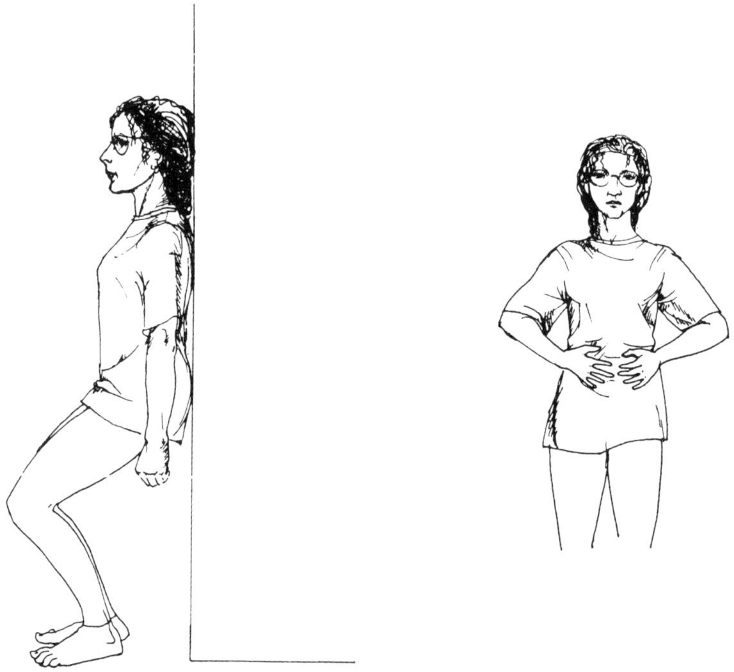

D—Wall Squats
E—Dynamic abdominal bracing

E. DYNAMIC ABDOMINAL BRACING

Place the hands on the waist and tighten your abdominal (tummy) muscles — do this by imagining you are gently drawing your belly button towards your back bone; cough gently to feel the abdominal muscle push out sideways. Hold for 20 seconds (don't forget to keep breathing while you count). Repeat 5 times. Also practise and use this whenever you are lifting anything.

(Devised by Mrs Sam Schirmer, Director of the Muscular Development Fitness Unit of the Memorial Hospital, Adelaide.)

Lawn Care

The English heritage of our 'Australian' gardening tradition is never so apparent as it is in our devotion to the lawn. The almost ubiquitous verdant spread fore and aft our homes is seen as a necessary part of the garden by many Australians, despite the high maintenance required in its upkeep. A turf lawn must be watered, fed, aerated and, above all, mown with regularity; how often these tasks will need to be done will depend on the weather, the soil type, the species of grasses grown and the inclinations of the gardener. But whether these jobs pan out to once a week or once a year, one thing is true for all grass lawns—they will require regular mowing *ad infinitum*—they are absolutely relentless in this regard. Consequently, it is important that gardeners who like a bit of a lawn (and I am one of them) have some painless means of keeping their grass cut. Having your lawn mown professionally is an option which is becoming more and more popular with Australian gardeners, but if you opt for cutting it yourself, make sure you have a good, reliable mower that is easy to use, effective, comfortable to work with, and *safe*.

Choosing a lawn-mower

There are a number of questions to ask yourself when choosing a lawn-mower. They include the following:

(a) Does the mower start readily in *your* hands? Some gardeners may opt for an electric mower in order to avoid the gut-busting business of starting a petrol-driven mower. Be aware that electric mowers require two hands to start them—one to push the safety lock button, and one to hold down the lever poetically known as the 'deadman's handle'. As a safety feature, the mower will only operate while this hand lever is depressed, so if the handle is released, the power is cut and the motor stops.

(b) Is the mower powerful enough to cut *your* lawn? A lawn that is kept short will be easier to cut than long, rank grasses. Petrol-driven mowers cut long grass better than the electric mowers currently available, although the electric mowers are more than able to cut any reasonably well maintained lawn.

(c) Is the mower comfortable for *you* to mow with? Are the handles at a comfortable height, is the mower sufficiently light? Handles may adjust automatically to your height (known as 'floating handles') or they may offer a choice of heights. A petrol mower must be pushed along, while electric mowers may be of either the 'hover' variety or it may run on wheels. Electric mowers are generally easier to use than petrol; however, when the hover-types are not running, they must be picked up and carried in order to move them. This may not suit everyone, especially those gardeners who have some distance between their storage facilities and their lawn. Electric mowers cause less vibration than petrol models, which may make a big difference to some gardeners.

(d) Is the mower safe for *you* to use? With electric mowers, the long power lead which is necessary to run the mower can often get itself tangled or get caught on trees and so forth, which can cause a lot of to-ing and fro-ing. Then, too, there is the danger of running over the extension lead during a lapse in concentration, thereby cutting through the lead. If you are likely to find such things a problem, then take this into account when making your choice. Although electric mowers are well insulated, if you opt for one, make sure you use it with an electrical safety switch—either a portable one, or one fitted permanently on your electricity meter. Don't use an electric mower in the rain, and don't let the lead go anywhere near water, ponds and swimming pools included. Doing either of these will put you at risk of electrocution. Read the manufacturer's instructions carefully and follow their recommendations. Check, too, that the blade is properly guarded so that it is not possible to put your foot into the blade when it is rotating.

Both electric and petrol driven mowers are noisy, and ultimately they all add to pollution. If you are hale and hearty, have a small lawn with well maintained, easy to cut grass, you may well prefer to use a hand-mower. However, unless these three conditions are satisfied, mowing a lawn with a hand-mower is going to be a little too much like hard work. If you find using a power mower unacceptable, but a hand-mower impractical, then perhaps you should consider alternatives to a grass lawn, such as paving or non-grass plants. These are discussed in later chapters.

When choosing a mower, it is perhaps wise to first consult a consumer advice magazine such as *Choice*. These are usually held by local and State libraries and are a valuable first step in the selection process. Although the magazines can only survey most things every few years, they are nevertheless a good guide to reliable manufacturers and general issues in choosing an appliance.

Having arrived at a short-list of sorts, visit a display centre of a stockist to see which of these mowers you find easy to start and comfortable to run before making your final choice. I would suggest you use a retailer that specialises in mowers for this last step, particularly one which also does repairs. The large hardware stores often do not know as much about their stock as is desirable, and furthermore, they will have no idea about any common problems that may arise once the guarantee has expired. Although a smaller retailer may charge a little more for an item, their greater product knowledge makes it worthwile, and they are usually willing to take some responsibility for a mower they have sold you, should anything go wrong.

Protective clothing

Always wear suitable clothing when using a mower. Take a look at workers of a professional lawn mowing service—you will find them clad in heavy boots, safety goggles, as well as gloves and ear muffs. Follow their example—closed in shoes and safety goggles are an absolute minimum requirement, and don't forget a hat when the sun is shining.

Edging the lawn

Edging a lawn can be a fiddly business, but one which can be neglected for only so long. Edging can be done using a variety of different hand tools, ranging from short-handled grass shears to whizz-bang electrical gadgets. In the youthful enthusiasm of my thirties and early forties, I would get down on my hands and knees and trim the edging using hand shears (in China, I am told, whole armies of workers cut entire lawns using hand shears!) however, it is not a method I would recommend.

There are a number of tools made for edging the lawn while in a standing position. These include rotary edgers and half moon cutting edgers. These are available on long handles from the mainstream manufacturers, and edging tool-heads are also available in the multi-change tool range. All do the job well in the right hands, and again, it is personal preference which determines just which edger will serve a gardener best. Long-handled shears with the blades set at right angles to the handle shafts are also available. Known as border shears and lawn shears, these odd looking tools resemble nothing so much as the flamingos used as croquet mallets by the Queen of Hearts in *Alice in Wonderland*, but actually do the job rather well. (See photo 42.)

Motorised lawn trimmers, which are often known by the brand name 'Whipper Snipper', are often used successfully as lawn edgers. There are both petrol and electric trimmers available. Again, the electric versions are considerably lighter than the petrol-powered version but they are less useful with longer grass. The same steps and selection criteria should be applied to trimmers as to mowers (see above), and the same safety precautions should be taken when using them. Power edgers are also available.

Additional Safety Issues

Power tools

There is a wealth of power tools now available for the home gardener—hedge trimmers, edge cutters, munchers that chew up your prunings and spit out mulch; there are garden vacuums, garden blowers, garden vac-blowers—you name it, they've got it! These tools can save you a lot of work; if you're the type of gardener who enjoys electrical gadgetry, you may even get some positive pleasure out of using them. However, power tools are usually heavy, they vibrate when used, make a lot of noise, sometimes belch out filthy fumes and without exception contribute to pollution. There is also the potential for a nasty accident with any power tool. Always follow the manufacturer's safety instructions and do not use tools for anything other than the tasks they were designed for; do not attempt to trim your hedges with the electric mower, or prune your roses with the hedge clippers. The images these misuses conjure up may be amusing, but some rather grisly accidents have resulted from them.

Make sure you have sufficient strength to manage a power tool when in action before even contemplating using it. Often they are heavy enough when simply held; when in use, dealing with the vibrations, as well as any resistance from the material they are cutting through, can make them very difficult to control. Rechargeable battery-run tools are a little lighter, but there is a limited range of these available.

As with lawn-mowers, always wear appropriate protective clothing when using power tools. Closed-in shoes, gloves and safety goggles are mandatory.

Safety with garden sprays

Always take the necessary safety precautions when using any sprays in the garden. Rubber gloves and a face mask are the bare minimum and should always be worn *at all times* when using garden chemicals, particularly when working with the concentrates. Wear protective clothing when spraying all but the mildest of substances; pay particular attention to your footwear for you may well find yourself stepping into the spray as it settles—gumboots are a good idea. If you get any spray on your clothing, change them as soon as you are finished and make sure they are washed thoroughly before wearing them again.

Never spray on a windy day; not only is your spray likely to miss its mark, there is also a strong likelihood that you will find yourself covered in the spray, while your neighbours may find themselves the unwilling recipients of your chemical attentions. Never spray when there are any animals in the vicinity, and take care not to spray near ponds or waterways.

While some herbal sprays such as pyrethrum and garlic have been used safely for centuries, never lose sight of the fact that some of the most powerful poisons known are found in nature. When using naturally occurring chemicals, unless they come with a long history of safe usage, treat them with the same caution and respect that you would a synthetic chemical. Always wear rubber gloves and a face mask when working with concentrates, no matter how safe you may feel the substance to be.

If a spray cannot be stored when diluted, try to make up only as much spray as you need on that occasion. Unused garden chemicals should never be disposed of in normal household garbage collections; this can lead to seepage of the chemicals at the tip site, possibly resulting in long-term land contamination and pollution of our waterways. Nor should the unused sprays be tipped into household stormwater or sewerage systems or directly into waterways; the reasons for this are obvious with the more toxic substances, but even a relatively benign chemical, if present in large amounts, can upset a fragile ecosystem or destroy the bacteria used to purify the water at water treatment plants.

Safety with stakes

There are some plants that need a little extra support, such as carnations, large-flowered dahlias and the taller varieties of delphinium. If you are more concerned with creating a beautiful garden than in producing perfect specimens, then you will probably be content with growing these floppers in between firmer plants that will hold them up. If you want your perfect specimens, then you will probably insist on staking.

The most commonly used stakes are fine wood or bamboo. These often blend in with the plant so well that it is possible to forget that they are there, and it is all too easy to catch a tender portion of our persons upon their sharp little tips. The risk to eyes is actually quite great, especially for gardeners whose vision is already reduced. If you must stake, consider covering the tip of the stakes with something that is both conspicuous and non-sharp. I have seen empty soft drink cans and plastic pill bottles used for this, and while the visual effect may not be wonderful, at least the gardeners in question will not be putting their eyes out on the stakes. Wine corks are a more attractive alternative to pill bottles, though the stakes must be firmly driven into the corks to ensure that they remain in place.

Smaller shrubs and perennials can be staked safely using the wire hoops that are sold as garden edging (see photo 45). These 'hoop stakes' effectively restrain a plant while being both discreet and, more importantly, safe.

So take a good, hard look at your gardening tools. Are they serving you as well as they should, or is it perhaps time to invest in some new ones that are better suited to your changing needs as you adapt your gardening for retirement?

4
Gardening Methods that Save You Work

SOME GARDENING TASKS ARE A JOY TO PERFORM. WHICH TASKS A GARDENER enjoys is a matter of individual taste and what one gardener adores another abhors. There are, though, a number of tasks that most people regard as genuine chores—weeding is the one that springs instantly to mind. There are also some tasks which we may have enjoyed in the vigour of our younger gardening days but which become more and more demanding as we age; digging and heavy pruning fall into this group. Added to this is the fact that some of the horticultural practices commonly used are not only unnecessary but ultimately create more work than if they had been left undone. I place anything that disturbs the soil structure or which generally works against nature into this category.

The garden which requires the least labour is that which requires the least remedial action, that is, the least watering and weeding, spraying programs and fertiliser regimens. A garden in which each plant is placed with due regard for its requirements for light and moisture, its preferred (micro)climate and soil type, has every chance of flourishing. A soil left

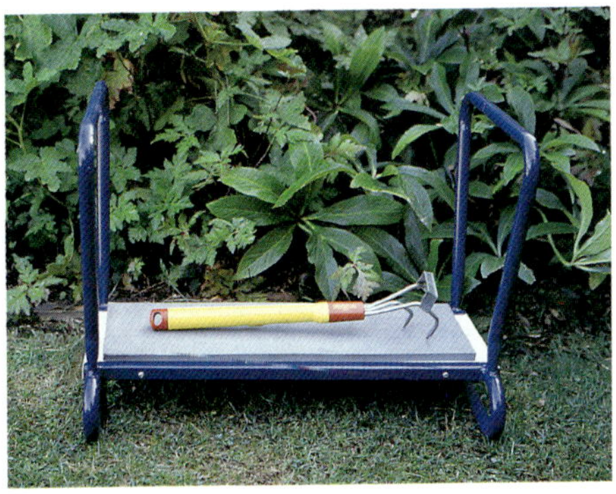

19

Kneeling Frame and short-handled tool

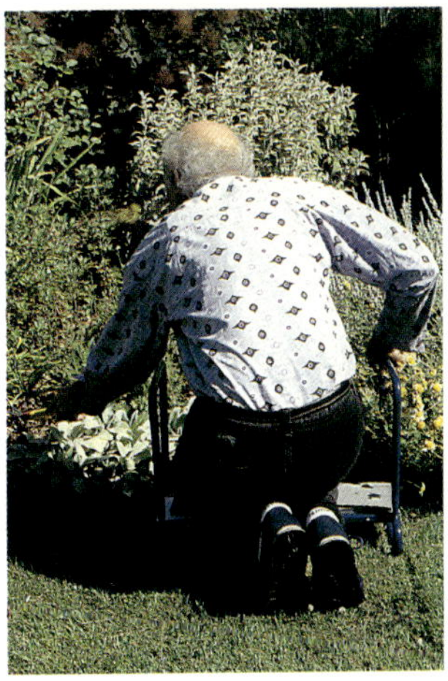

20

Kneeling Frame in use as a kneeler

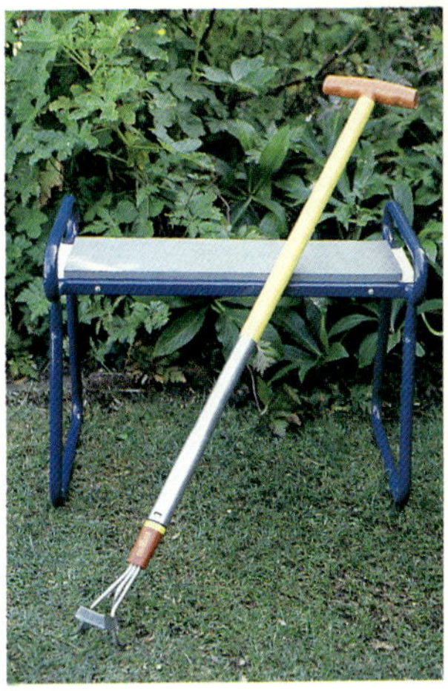

21

Kneeling Frame—this model inverts for use as a seat

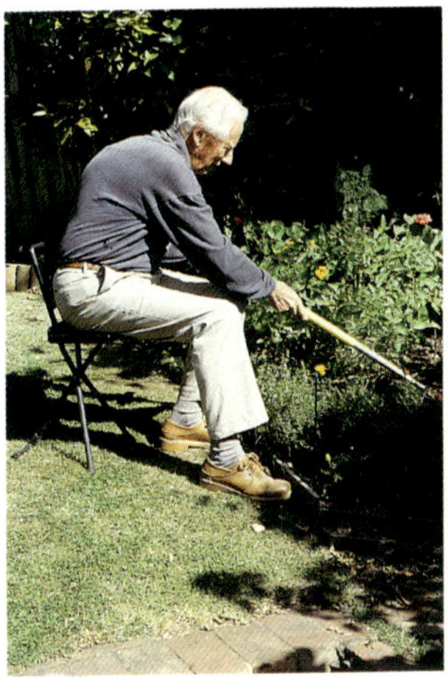

22

A portable golf-seat used as a garden work seat

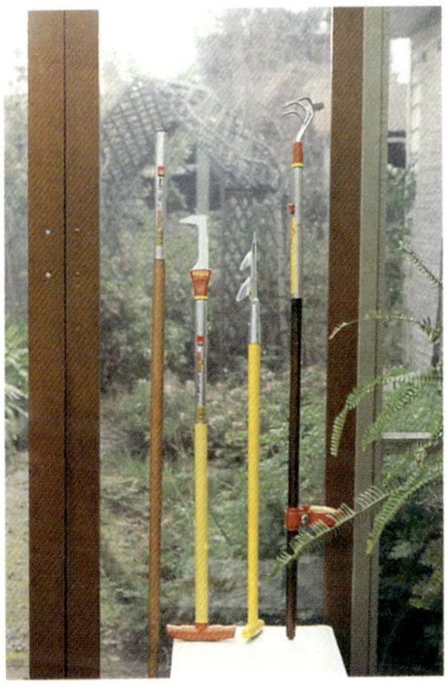

23

A selection of Wolf Tools *available with interchangable tool-heads, and handles of different lengths*

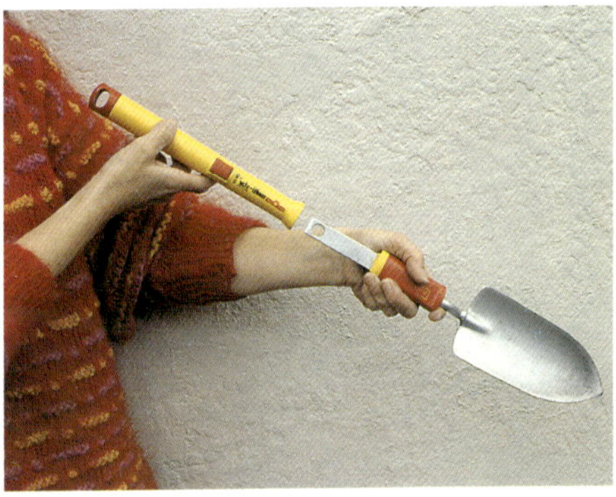

24

A close-up of the click-in system of the Wolf Tools

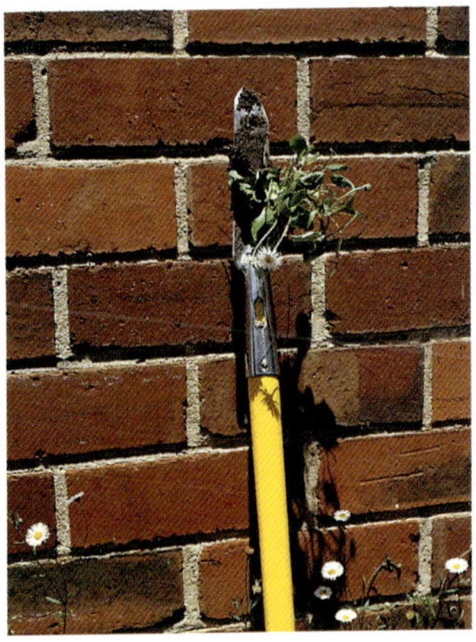

25

Harpoon Weeder *with a pulled lawn daisy*

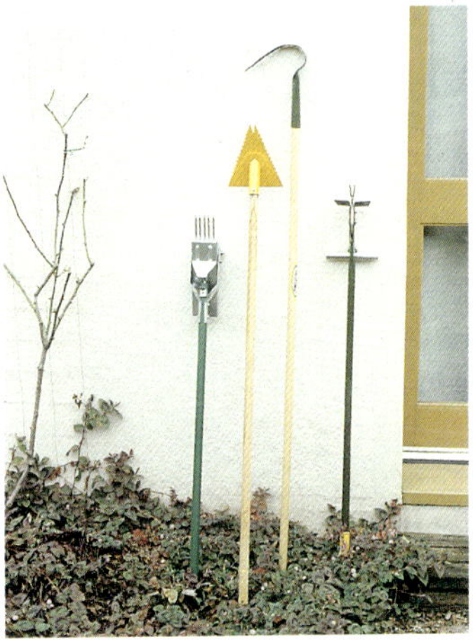

26

A selection of long-handled weeders

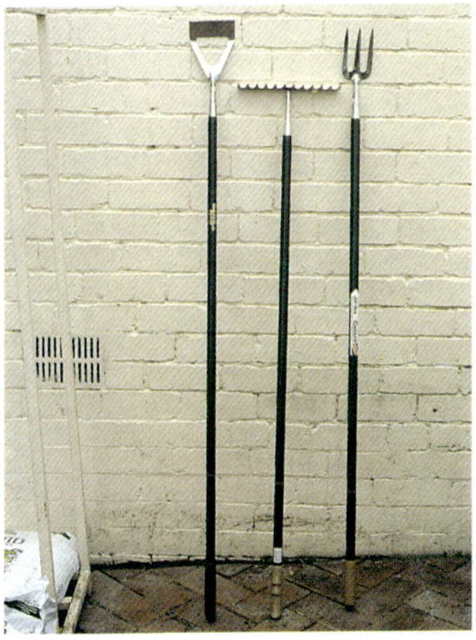

27

Small, light stainless steel tools

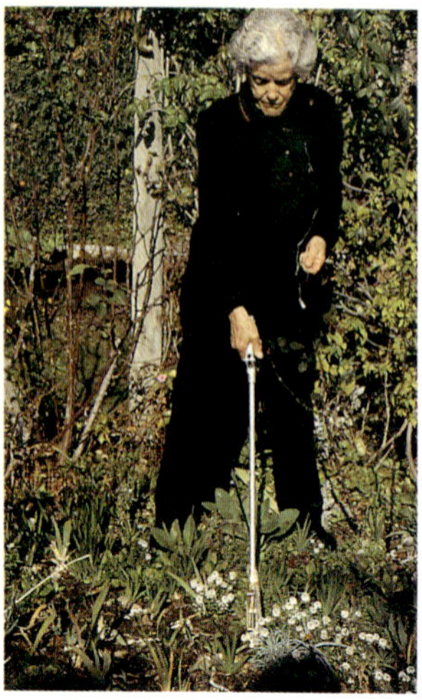

A trigger-operated weeder 28

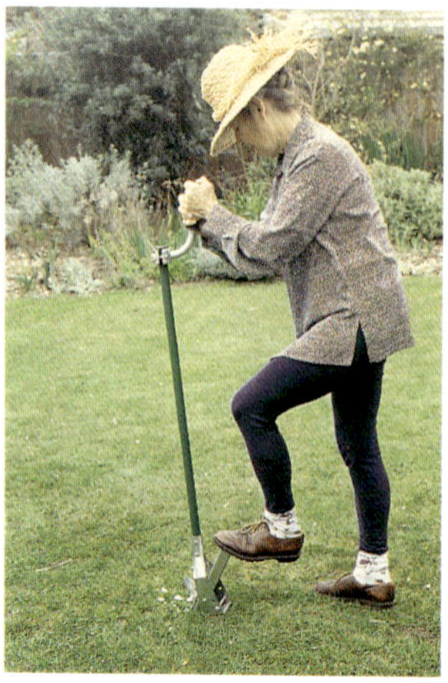

A pedal-operated weeder, extended with an Attach-A-Handle 29

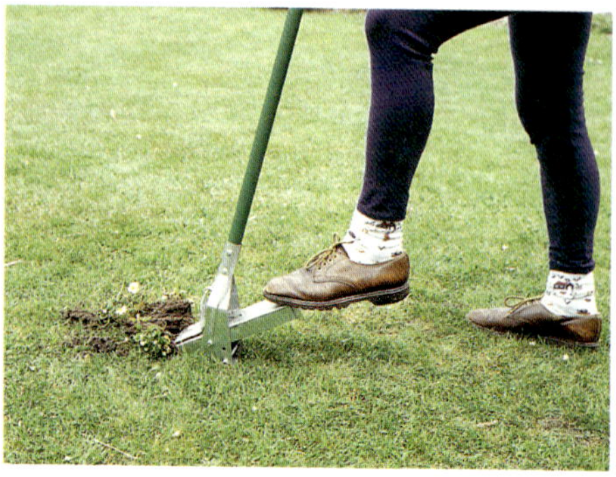

The foot-pedal operated weeder in action 30

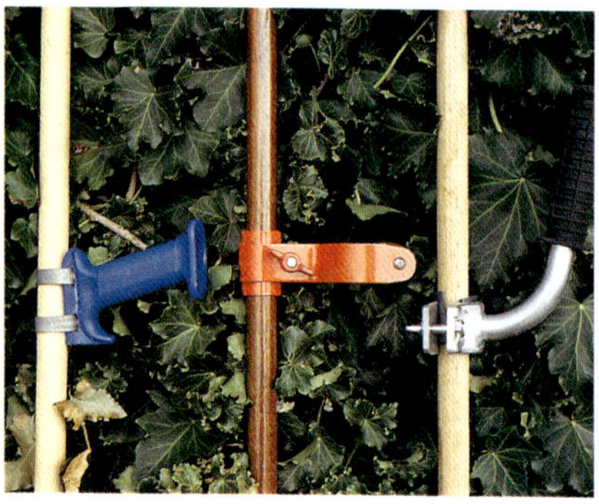

Auxilary handles 31

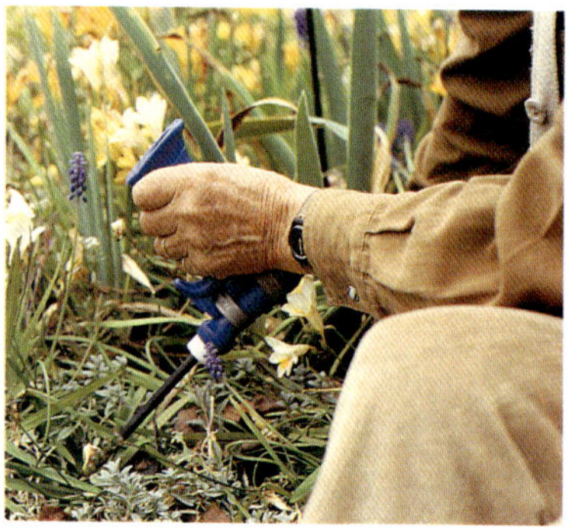

The Pistol-Grip Handle 32

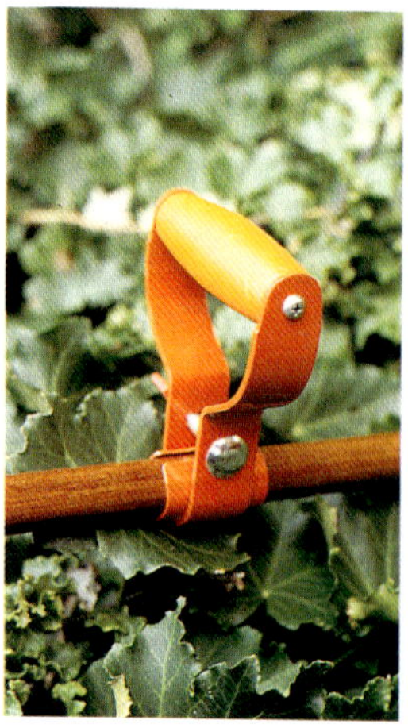

The Wolf *Auxiliary D-Handle* 33

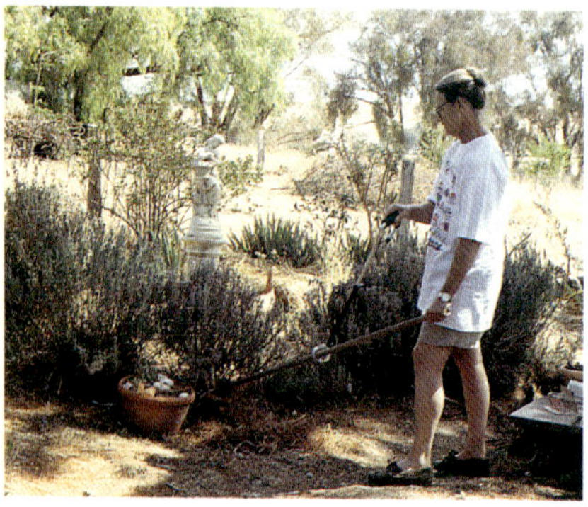

The Universal Back Saver 34

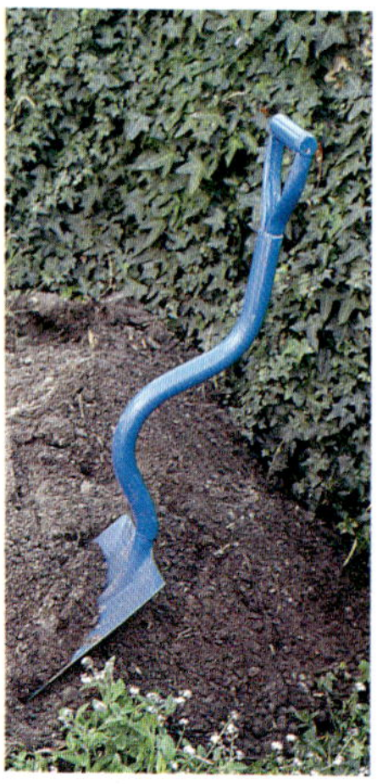

The Ergonomic Shovel 35

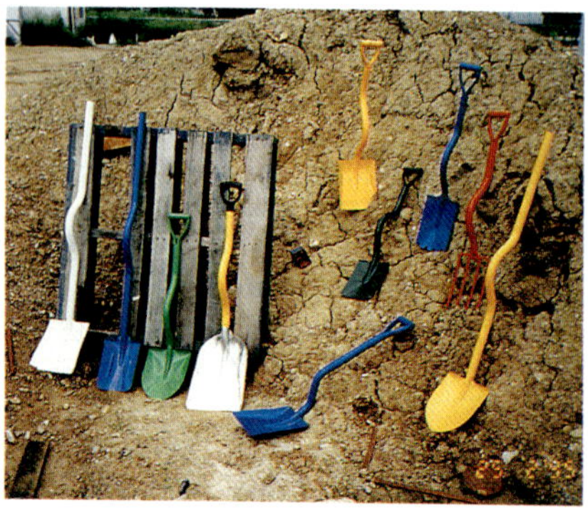

The range of Ergonomic tools 36

undisturbed by deep digging and given a protective cover of organic material is unlikely to be leached of nutrients, sprout weeds in vast numbers, dry out in the summer or sog up in the rains. Healthy plants will resist the ravages of disease and pests alike. By establishing a garden where nature is co-operated with rather than opposed, the gardener is creating an environment that will require minimal corrective intervention.

These contentions are not merely the rantings of an avid organic gardener, there are sound, scientific reasons why they are so to be found in the physiology of the plants and the structure of the soil. Plant growth and soil structure are given a bit of a scientific look-over at the end of this chapter. Many gardeners will be familiar with the information already, but those who are not, may find that a basic understanding of these can help sort out which gardening practices are sound and which are not (and might even make for an interesting read on a cold winter's night). Suffice it to say at this point that both a well-managed soil *and* growing conditions approximating those of the plant in its native environment are vital for its well-being. In particular, hold to your heart the maxim: 'For every dollar you spend on the plant, spend ten on the hole!' One of the ways we can best care for the soil is by mulching; by a happy stroke of fate, this practice also saves the gardener a great deal of hard labour.

Mulching

Mulching is the term used for covering the soil surface with a layer of material. Bare earth is like a wound; Nature seeks to heal that wound by whatever means it can—a cover of grasses, bushy regrowth, or a layer of leaf litter. Where this cannot occur, the cost is great—weed invasion, moisture imbalance, salting, erosion, soil degradation. The result of this abuse in work hours is immense, for garden or broad acre, but can be allayed by following nature's lead and covering the soil.

The main labour-saving benefits of mulching for the gardener are weed suppression and the prevention of water loss through surface evaporation. It is the single most labour-saving maintenance strategy that we can employ—I estimated that for every hour I spent mulching my garden in its early years, I saved myself two to three hours of back-breaking weeding, each week, every week through peak growing season. I seldom water my garden, even at the height of summer. While watering need not be either disagreeable or laborious if properly set up, both the financial and environmental aspects of water usage needs to be considered by all of us.

A variety of different materials can be used as mulch. Straw, pinebark, gravels and 'garden munchings', to mention a few will all suppress weeds and conserve moisture. They will also help to moderate soil temperatures, improve water penetration and prevent erosion. However, some will do some things better than others and some, the organic mulches, will bring additional benefits to your garden. Some have a further appeal in that they mimic the action of nature, for nature is constantly laying down dead or dying matter on the soil surface, be it leaf litter on the forest floor or spent annual grasses in the meadow. Organic mulches are excellent soil conditioners, improving the structure and adding to the nutrients as they decompose. The cost and availability will also be a consideration, as will be its appearance. An understanding of the way a mulch 'works' will allow you to make your selection according to what you want the mulch to achieve.

How a mulch works

Water conservation

A mulch will conserve existing moisture by preventing surface evaporation. The soil is held at a higher, more constant moisture level. Soils which would normally dry out in a few days will, when mulched, take several weeks to lose the same amount of water. Weeds can use as much water or even more than your garden plants and by suppressing weed growth a mulch will also prevent water being lost in this way. Condensation will occur on a cold mulch at night and so a permeable mulch can add this small amount of moisture to the soil as well. Mulches can also help to prevent the build-up of salt in the surface soil by slowing down the evaporation of water containing dissolved salts. This is an important consideration in many areas of the world where soil salinity has become a problem.

Weed suppression

Mulches suppress weeds by excluding the light that they need for growth. Weeds will not only compete with your garden plants for water, light and nutrients, some actually send substances into the soil that will damage young plants and prevent them from establishing properly.

Water penetration

A mulch will hold water near to where it has fallen, allowing the water to soak into the soil. An organic mulch will further increase water penetration by improving the soil structure.

Erosion reduction

By spreading the force of impact of rainfall or sprinkler drops, erosion of the surface soil is much reduced. By improving water penetration mulching also reduces run-off, another erosion-causing factor, and by providing a physical barrier at the soil surface a mulch will also protect against wind erosion.

Soil temperature moderation

A mulch will insulate the surface soil so that it is cooler in the summer and warmer in the winter than the bare soil. A mulched soil is slower to cool in the autumn, and slower to warm in the spring. This slower warming can delay the onset of spring growth and bud burst. While some authorities advise scraping back the mulch come spring, I view this delay as an asset, not a liability. After the mounting excitement then the pleasure of witnessing spring arrive in other peoples' gardens, I can enjoy an extended season in my own.

This insulating effect can be obtained using natural materials for the mulch layer—organic mulches, stones or gravel. Synthetic mulches such as black plastic sheeting are excellent barriers against weeds and water loss by surface evaporation; however, black plastic sheeting prevents both water and air from reaching the soil, and will raise the soil temperature to above that of its surroundings on a hot day. One study found that when the maximum daily temperature was 42°C (108°F) the bare soil reached 35° (95°F). None of the soils mulched with natural materials reached 30°, while the soil topped with black plastic topped 43°! Other synthetic mulches, though not quite cooking your soil like the plastic sheeting, also offer little in the way of insulation.

Organic mulches

By gradually decomposing and adding to the organic matter in the soil, an organic mulch will improve both the texture and the nutrient content of the soil (see 'Soil structure' at the end of this chapter). The soil will have a higher number of beneficial soil dwelling organisms. This will further increase the amount of organic matter and lead to improved porosity, hence improving water penetration and aeration.

Choice of mulching material

The first consideration when choosing a mulch is *what you want it to achieve in your garden*. For instance, you may live in a high rainfall area where the climate is mild, the soil structure is good and where you have found that a regime of liquid fertilisers suits your style of gardening. You will probably only be concerned with the weed-suppressing properties of a mulch. A man-made mulching material such as a woven plastic weed mat may fill your requirements. On the other hand, you may live in an area where your plants are baked in the summer heat and the soil is parched in long dry spells but where the soil structure is good and the supply of organic matter adequate. You will require a mulch that will provide some insulation from the heat and that will minimise surface evaporation as well as suppress the weeds; however, since the soil structure is sound, a mulch which breaks down relatively slowly while performing these other functions is an option. Wood chips or pine bark would be suitable in this case.

If you also need the mulch to contribute to the level of organic matter in the soil, then an organic mulch that decomposes over the course of a year would be a sound choice. Straw or garden 'munchings' are both suitable. The finer the particles of a given organic mulch, the more rapidly it will decompose. Be aware that certain organic materials such as leaf mould, rotted manures and compost, while doing wonders for your soil quality and water retention, do very little, if anything, to suppress the weeds.

Recently a felted wool mulching material rather like carpet underfelt has become available. It is completely organic and has all the above mentioned benefits of an organic mulch (soil improvement, water retention, temperature insulation, erosion control) combined with the weed suppressive properties of a sheet mulch. It can be bought in a range of weights; the heavier the mulch, the longer it will take to break down. The material is still being trialled in the field; however, I have found that the medium thickness does not last any longer than a mulch of old woollen carpet or an organic underfelt.

The woollen mulch is sold by the metre or in 60 cm squares; it is an excellent soil conditioner. It is very easy to lay on an empty garden bed, and is comparable in price to wood chips per square metre of soil mulched, although its appearance is improved by a cosmetic covering of some other mulching material which also helps to weight it down at the edges against the effects of the wind, the dog and marauding birds. The stockist is listed at the end of the book.

Availability and expense may also influence your choice. Some materials may be only locally available or else the cost of transport makes them prohibitively expensive outside the area in which they are produced. It can sometimes be difficult to locate a supplier for some of the more unusual mulches and unless word-of-mouth can lead you to a source, you may be limited to what is available through landscape suppliers in your area.

Some local councils are now producing garden 'munchings' from tree prunings and so forth from their parks and the street trees, then making them available to residents at a nominal cost. Your local 'Parks and Gardens' should be able to help you with information on this. You may prefer to produce your own mulch by grinding your own garden 'debris', such as prunings from trees and shrubs, fallen leaves and the like.

The appearance of a mulch may also be important. Some mulches have a strong visual character and may look amiss in some styles of garden. A straw mulch may not sit easily in a garden of Australian natives, at least not until it has weathered. A gravel mulch can appear harsh in a cottage garden while 'mulchings' can look a little casual in some formal settings. Newspaper is an excellent mulch if applied several sheets thick but its appearance leaves something to be desired. Often a happy compromise between conflicting considerations is achieved by combining differing mulching materials. A layer of four or five sheets of newspaper topped with a layer of more attractive but also more expensive mulch will cut down on cost without compromising either its function or its appearance.

A word of caution seems called for at this point. I have used newspaper in combination with straw in my vegetable garden at the front of the house, and with 'munchings' at the back for my ornamentals. At first, both of these combinations were successful, but at some stage the birds 'discovered' my garden. They came in hungry droves one winter, in quest of the earthworms to be found there in the warm, well-nourished soil beneath the mulch. That the particles of the 'munchings' were strewn everywhere and the soil exposed in patches I did not mind so much—these were easily put to rights with a long-handled garden sweep. It was the shreds of newspaper tossed high and low with wild abandon that I found wearing—caught in branches and scattered over the mulch, they created a bizarre, almost surreal effect in the winter landscape. Repairing the damage proved more than my patience would stand and after a repeat performance the following winter, I switched to using only 'munchings' on my ornamentals. Curiously, the newspaper under the straw in my front garden has escaped this fate so far, and I continue to use it without mishap in the vegie patch.

There has been some concern that mulching can lead to a decrease in available nitrogen at the soil surface. This has proved to be not the case with the vast majority of mulches. When it does occur it is short term and restricted to the topmost portion of the surface soil, above the layer where roots are found. Cautious gardeners may like to apply their preferred nitrogen source before mulching. I put down pelletised chicken manure below the mulch as a matter of course each year and find that this satisfies the needs of all but the grossest of feeders—please excuse the term!

How to put down a mulch

A mulch is not at all difficult to put down, but it takes a little forethought, and it must be done properly to gain maximum benefit.

Preparation—Weed eradication

Perennial weeds can grow through a mulch, especially those weeds with pointed tips such a couch grass and kikuyu, so it is important to clear these from your garden bed before you mulch. There are several ways to do this.

Hand weeding This is the simplest method and the one that has the most immediate effect. However, if a large amount of weeding is involved, or if you find hand weeding difficult, then an alternative method should be used. It is important to lay down a mulch soon after you have cleared the ground to avoid any more weeds germinating in the bare soil. At any one time, clear only that area that you are sure you can mulch within the next few days.

Herbicides Some gardeners will be unhappy at the thought of using any non-naturally occuring chemicals in the garden. Indeed, I generally fall into that category myself; however, the Glyphosate-based herbicides which are sold under various brand names, including Zero and Round-Up, do seem to be safe. The Glyphosate is applied directly to the weeds, but any that reaches the soil binds quickly to the soil particles, thus causing no problems with run-off, and breaking down after only a short time. It has been used in a number of environmentally sensitive areas and has had no observed ill effects. The Glyphosate is sprayed onto the foliage of the offending weeds, where it is taken up into the plant. Once inside, Glyphosate does its damage by killing the plant from the roots up. The top of the plant turns yellow about two weeks after applying the spray, by which time the roots are well and truly dead. Care must be taken not to get the chemical on your garden plants—Glyphosate does not differentiate between weeds and non-weeds but kills both with equal efficiency.

Care should also be taken with your own safety. Again, always wear rubber gloves and a mask as well as solid shoes when using garden chemicals, no matter how safe they seem.

A 'weed wand' is available for dabbing the Glyphosate accurately on isolated weeds, as is a spray applicator with an inverted-funnel style hood covering the spray outlet to keep it from wandering beyond its intended target. Both these applicators have handles of around 1 metre long—this allows the application of the herbicide with minimum bending. The applicator with the hooded outlet may well prove useful for general weeding purposes.

Mechanical means Cultivation is a time-honoured method of clearing the soil of weeds. Whether done with a hand-held tool or a power driven rotary hoe, cultivation will disrupt the soil structure, and I hope to dissuade you from doing so in your garden in a later section on no-dig gardens. A weed is usually more than just a 'plant in the wrong place'. For a plant to establish itself in large enough numbers to become a nuisance, it must have some kind of advantage over other plants. Often, this is due to highly efficient reproductive strategies; one such strategy is to set a huge amount of seed that can germinate for many, many years after, providing the conditions are right. Whenever the soil is cultivated, some of these seeds are brought to the surface and given just the conditions they need to start growing—that is why a newly turned over bed of fertile soil will sprout a rash of weeds in no time. But if these seeds are kept buried, they'll never even get a look in. Moreover, there are a number of perennial weeds that will regenerate from even the tiniest piece. Cultivation will cut these weeds up into many smaller bits, all of which will grow to be an entire new plant, thus giving a far greater weed problem than there was in the first place.

Applying the mulch—For the well-being of your plants

Before laying the mulch on the soil, make sure that the garden is well-watered, if necessary giving it a good soak before starting. If you are applying mulch made up of separate particles, such as pine bark or garden munchings, try distributing it by tossing it over your garden, either in handfuls or in small bucketfuls. A layer of around 10 cm (4″) is needed with most mulches. Too little will let the light in, let the moisture out and offer proportionally less insulation. Too deep a layer can be detrimental too, so it is best to stick to a happy medium.

If using an expensive mulch such as wood chips or pine bark combined with a bottom layer of newspaper, then you can reduce the amount of top mulch in accordance with the amount of newspaper used. With a full measure of 8–10 sheets only a cosmetic cover of the other mulch is needed. If a half measure of 4–5 sheets of newspaper is used, then a half measure of top mulch will be needed.

It is important not to pack the top mulch up against the stems or trunks of plants or else collar rot can result. If mulching in the winter when some plants have died back above the surface, mark their places and do not cover with mulch, or they may not emerge to greet you in the spring!

Water well again after laying an organic mulch; since the mulch will absorb a certain amount of water itself, make sure that you start off with it thoroughly wetted right through. It will also help the mulch to settle down and start the weathering process that will allow it to blend in visually with the garden.

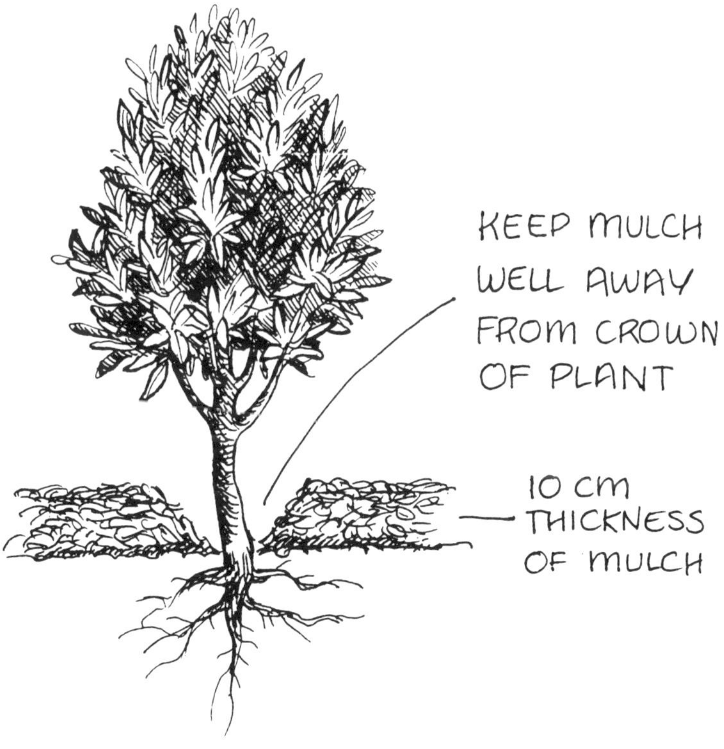

A well-mulched plant.

Applying the mulch—For the well-being of your back

Pacing yourself If you have a garden 'muncher' you are likely to mulch as you go, making and distributing the munching as the raw materials become available. This lends itself naturally to pacing, a good principle to observe in the garden no matter what you are doing. Those gardeners who must buy in mulch are faced with a great pile of it arriving all at once, and it is difficult not to feel pressurised by its presence. Unless the pile causes problems of access, safety or security, try to approach the task with a 'Tortoise and the Hare' philosophy. If the mulch really *must* be moved in one hit, then perhaps it's time to invite your friends and family to a bring-a-barrow bring-a-plate picnic mulch-in. Try to shift the mulch using whatever tool allows you to do this with minimum physical strain. Refer to the previous chapter on tools if in doubt on this score.

Choosing the right tools When distributing the mulch, move the material to its intended home in a lightweight pull-along wheelbarrow or even a laundry trolley. The latter choice is particularly good if you need to minimise bending (see photo 46). The laundry basket sits higher than does the barrow, making it an easy matter to scoop up the mulch in a bucket or bowl, or to empty the whole basket onto the garden if this is comfortable for you. Pine bark, munchings and other mulches consisting of smallish particles can be distributed about the garden just by tossing. I find that the upper parts of low growing plants prevent most of the mulch from landing too near the crown. Once on the garden, it is an easy job to shift the mulch around using a long-handled garden sweep or even a small fork. If using a baled mulch such as straw you will find that it is often packed into the bales in 'cakes'; these cakes can be conveniently lifted off and laid down whole. If you wish to avoid bending, the straw can be thrown down and then placed more exactly in the desired spot using a long-handled tool. A 'Garden Gripper' (see photo 44) is useful for doing this and in fact can be used to perform the entire operation, lifting the straw from the bale onto the garden.

A garden gripper can be used as well to put down a mulch of newspaper. A word of warning here—avoid windy days for this task or you will spend all your time *chasing* the newspaper instead of mulching with it. Dampen the newspaper as you go, laying a wad at a time, and then lightly water it. This will stop it lifting if a breeze does blow up—as it invariably seems to when one is mulching—but get the top mulch onto it as soon as possible to weight it down.

Living mulches

Groundcovers

Planting close together so that the leaves of adjacent plants are touching will obviously cover the ground, so depriving the weeds of exposed soil in which to germinate. Gardeners are often advised to use a planting of 'groundcovers' to suppress the weeds. A 'groundcover' is usually seen as a low growing plant, but in fact a groundcover can be any plant that grows in such a way that it will shade the soil. There are a huge number of plants that fit this description and gardeners can find plants of a range of heights to suit any climate, soil type or gardening style. See Chapter 6 for some suggestions.

If you are putting in ground covers to escape the effects of competition from the weeds, be aware that ground covers have their own requirements for water, light and nutrients. It is important to match the requirements of the ground cover to both the site *and* the existing planting. It may be possible to exploit a niche that the rest of your garden has created, for example, a shade-loving ground cover could be planted in the shade created by a neighbouring shrub, a drough-tolerant prostrate native could be planted at the top of a bank of indigenous species that have a slightly higher water requirement. By and large, though, planting a ground cover with a different water requirement to the rest of the planting is definitely not a good idea: it will lead to complicated watering regimes and/or unhappy plants.

Cover crops

Cover crops are used in some agricultural systems where compatible crops are grown together. The technique is easily scaled down for the home garden. Usually the main crop is grown with a secondary 'crop which improves the soil composition after its decomposition or which protects the crop in some way; some cover crops do both. These methods are often a radical departure from conventional agricultural practices. For the last forty years, scientist turned farmer, Masanobu Fukuoko, has been using the annual white clover as a cover crop for rice and other grains. He has devised a no-tillage system that mimics nature and is very different from that used to grow rice in flooded paddy fields; he has extended the technique to vegetable crops and orchard trees. The CSIRO have developed a similar system using a winter growing perennial clover whose aboveground parts die down in the summer. Summer crops are planted out *into* the clover in spring. As the main crops grow up the clover leaves brown off and die, providing all the benefits of an organic mulch as they rot down. In the following winter, the underground parts of the clover spring into action and the leaves shoot again.

Anyone interested in cover crops or no-tillage gardens may be interested to read Fukuoko's *The One Straw Revolution*, or his more recent *The Natural Way of Farming*. *Permaculture II* by Bill Mollison has a section on no-tillage cropping and an extensive list of further reading.

No-Dig Gardening

A number of systems have evolved around the world that allow us to enjoy bountiful gardens without the back-breaking labour of digging. Many gardeners feel that digging is a vital part of garden-making; if this is so of you and you find it therapeutic without doing you any damage then far be it from me to interfere! However, please be aware that you are damaging your soil each time you turn it over. A look at why we have traditionally dug the soil and what we hope to achieve by doing so would seem timely. An awareness of what digging actually does may bring a change of heart towards this time-honoured practice.

Soil is traditionally turned to 'open it up' and so improve aeration and water infiltration and to allow the roots to grow through with ease. It is also done to incorporate whatever it is felt the soil is lacking. Let us examine both of these in turn.

Aeration and water penetration are both improved by the presence of continuous soil spaces. These continuous pores also offer the optimal conditions for root activity and other biological processes. An uncultivated soil is more likely to have continuous pores. Digging disrupts this continuity and damages the plant roots which have been stabilising the structure. Soil may be 'fluffed up' after turning but because it has been destablised it is very prone to compaction. Turning the soil also buries the fertile top a few centimeters beyond the immediate reach of young plant roots.

Many gardeners already maintain their permanent planting by no-dig strategies. Trees and shrubs will suffer if their roots are damaged by digging; an annual top dressing of fertiliser before the main growth period, followed by a layer of mulch is sufficient for most woody plants. It is in growing annual crops that no-dig gardening is most innovative and saves us real hard yakka. The following method is the one that I use for my own vegetable plot. It is a synthesis of things that I have read, been told, overhead, misheard and worked out for myself. I have used this method to set up and maintain my kitchen garden for a number of years now in the centre of the lawn in my suburban front yard.

Setting up a no-dig garden involves smothering the existing vegetation with a sheet mulch, then providing a top layer of nutrient-rich material in which to grow your plants. In my no-dig garden, nitrogen-rich organic matter is first laid down under the sheet mulch. I use a sheet mulch layer (of either cardboard or newspaper) that is thick enough to suppress the lawn but which will still allow the crop plants—both annual and perennial—to eventually put their roots down into the soil. This allows me to take advantage of the good soil structure that exists (as is usually the case) under the uncompacted lawn.

This sheet mulch is then topped with either fresh or dried manure and then with a mulch of pea straw. Seeds are sown or seedlings planted into mounds of compost within the pea straw to start them off. As the straw rots down, aided by the manure, it provides a rich growing medium for the plants. The materials that I use are those that I find convenient and easy to obtain and which do not offend suburban sensibilities. Substitute your own selections where they will do the same job at less cost, greater convenience or increased aesthetic appeal.

If your soil underneath is in poor condition, vary the formula by adding a deeper layer of straw; plant your seedling into a correspondingly larger mound of compost. This will ensure that the young plants will have sufficient 'soil' to grow into as the straw rots down. The soil underneath will be greatly improved as successive layers of mulch rot down and you should be able to reduce your mulch layers with time. Here is my recipe for setting up a no-dig garden:

1. Mark out the area you wish to use for your garden. A border of wooden planks or bricks will make maintenance easier but it is not really necessary.

2. Sprinkle nitrogen-rich organic matter on top of the area. I use pelletised manure but you can substitute Blood and Bone or fresh manure. This encourages various beneficial soil-dwelling organisms into the area where they commence improving the soil immediately on arrival. An added dollop of organic matter, such as fallen leaves, lawn clippings or hedge prunings, when laid down here will enhance their activity; I seldom have a supply on hand and I find that the soil is soon 'jumping' anyway.

3. Lay down a sheet mulch of cardboard and/or newspaper to completely cover the area. I use old cardboard boxes flattened out or else newspaper laid 10 sheets thick. If you are concerned about the more vigorous creeping weeds such as couch grass or kikuyu, consider spraying the area first with Glyphosate weed killer. Allow time for the spray to work before proceeding with the next step—ten to fourteen days will usually see the leaves yellowing, and by this time the roots will already be dead. Make sure there are no gaps for weeds to poke through—overlap the papers a little. Again, avoid windy days for the task, and dampen down the paper as you go.

4. Sprinkle more nitrogen-rich fertiliser on top of the sheet mulch. Again I used pelletised manure.

5. Top with a 15 cm (6″) layer of straw. I find that a crop of seedling 'straw' plants is inevitable with all straws. I use pea straw because the crop of pea seedlings is easier to remove than the seedlings of other types of straw. Again it is a matter of personal preference—a layer of lucern hay is also recommended and is preferred by some gardeners. Do not use wheat or oaten straw in this layer or you will soon have a lawn of germinating seedlings within your mulch.

6. Part the straw and place mounds of compost within the straw layer. I make little hillocks of compost about 15 cm (6″) deep and the same across if I am planting seedlings or sowing large seeds. I form a long ridge of compost also of 15 cm depth if I am sowing fine seed. (I find that root crops prefer deeper layers of straw and compost.) Plant or sow into the compost as you would into the soil. Pull the parted mulch back to almost reach the plant or seed/s. Water well. (See photos 50–52).

Setting up a no-dig garden does take a little time and effort but compares favourably with a conventional vegetable garden. It takes me about 20 minutes and two-thirds of a bale of straw to set up a bed of 1.2 metres by 1.2 metres (4′x4′). I top up the manure and the straw as necessary throughout the year and re-lay the whole thing anew each spring on top of the old mulch. Perennial residents of my vegetable patch, such as rhubarb, french sorrell and various culinary herbs are mulched *around* each spring. Newspaper is drawn up as close as possible to each plant, then covered in straw. For closely planted rows it is only necessary to mulch with straw between established plants.

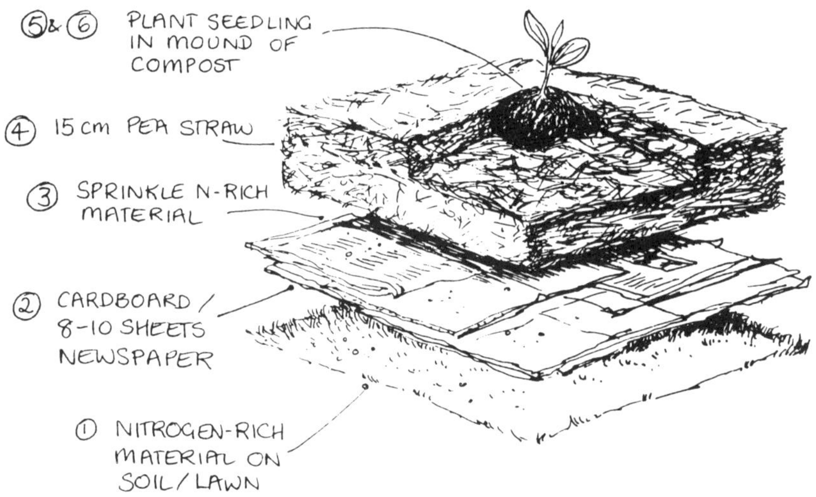

A '*No-Dig*' garden.

This method can also be adapted for use as a method of preparing a garden bed. A thick layer of fresh organic material and manure beneath the sheet mulch will speed up the improvement of the soil underneath. The rate of this soil improvement will depend on a number of factors such as the prevailing temperatures, the state of the soil and the type and the amount of the organic material. After setting up the bed, seedlings and young plants can be planted out in compost in the upper mulch as before. By the time the straw has rotted down to ground level the soil underneath may well have softened sufficiently for it to be planted directly into. If, after checking, you feel it needs to 'cook' for a little longer, top it up with extra manure and mulch and leave for a further period.

A No-Dig garden can also be set up over concrete or rocky ground. To do this, place a drainage layer between the ground and the sheet mulch—a layer of sticks or gravel is suitable for this. Obviously there is no question of soil improvement here; plant growth must be provided for entirely by the upper mulch layers.

Easy-Reach Fruit Trees

One of the most keenly savoured pleasures of the home garden for many of us is producing our own fruit. To eat a fragrant, sun-ripened fruit plucked straight from the tree can be a truly memorable experience. Home-grown fruit is often of superior taste and texture to that which has been commercially produced, and those who grow organically have the benefit of knowing that there are no damaging chemicals in their produce. As well, many varieties of fruit can be grown at home which are not to be found in commercial nurseries. All gardeners who grow their own fruit have the satisfaction of providing at least in part for their own needs and of reaping a tangible reward for their labours.

Fruit tree maintenance is highly seasonal. By and large, the gardener can forget about their fruit trees and let nature just get on with it. However, come harvest time there must be many a gardener, young and old, who wishes that their trees were a little bit smaller. Fruit borne high on a large-grown tree often proves inaccessible to humans, though alas not so to the birds. Netting against birds becomes impractical, harvesting becomes an ordeal. How much more sensible to grow trees of a compact and accessible form. One need not even resign oneself to a lower yield; a number of commercial orchards are now finding that they obtain a better yield by growing a larger number of dwarf trees in the space where they previously grew full-sized trees. Come pruning time, the wisdom of having low-growing trees will again be apparent. The pruning needs of a tree with a canopy that is easily reached from the ground will be met with minimum inconvenience.

There are three main ways of obtaining small-growing trees. The first means is by using trees that will only grow to the desired height. Secondly, the overall size of the plant can be limited by restricting the spread of the roots. Finally, the canopy of the tree—that is, the parts above the trunk (the branches) can be trained to conform to the desired dimensions. Let us consider each in turn.

Dwarf fruit trees

A dwarf tree may be a genetic dwarf—that is, one which is naturally small-growing, or it may be the result of having been grafted onto special dwarfing root stock. A dwarfing root stock will limit the overall size of the tree. In both cases the amount of fruit that the tree will bear will be proportionately reduced although the quality and the size of the fruit will be unaffected.

There are few genetic dwarves among fruit trees. In Australia at present only peach and nectarine genetic dwarves are available. Growing to around 1.5 metres (5′) in height, these trees are grown mainly for the ornamental value of their blossom. The peach trees (which, incidentally, can be obtained in a choice of blossom colour) produce sweet fruit of a good flavour but which bruise easily—you have to be standing there ready to catch the fruit as it ripens! The dwarf nectarine is more satisfactory as a fruiting tree. The yellow-fleshed fruit has a good flavour and is not especially prone to bruising.

Apple trees on dwarfing rootstock are readily available and have been for some time. Some citrus plants are also available dwarfed. In European countries there is a great interest in fruit grown on dwarfing root stock and a wider range of dwarfed trees is available there than we have in this country at present. In Australia, until recently the nursery trade has had little demand for smaller trees—residential land has not been in short supply; older members of our society have had little voice, nor have they often thought to ask. There has been little reason for nurseries to embark on the long and costly process of importation and the subsequent research and development.

Introducing a new plant line requires an enormous investment of time, energy, and money on the part of the nurseries; at the outset they do not know if they will ever receive any return for their investment and may have to wait for over a decade to find out. Land in developed areas is now at a premium; more and more of us find ourselves living, and gardening, in smaller spaces. With our burgeoning 'grey' population, more attention is being paid to the needs of older people. These factors have made some of the larger nurseries aware of the advantages of producing dwarfed trees. They are currently trialling dwarfing root stocks for compatibility with locally-grown varieties and suitability for local conditions. Hopefully we will see an increase in the number of varieties of dwarfed trees available over the next decade or two.

Root restriction

Anything that restricts the size of the roots of a plant will restrict the size of the above ground parts—this is the principle of Bonsai. Plants which would grow to substantial sized trees are manipulated in such a way that they grow to perhaps only a handspan in height. This is achieved by pruning the roots of the tree at regular time intervals and by restricting the plant to a tiny container from the time it was a seedling. Such drastic measures may have little application in the home garden but they demonstrate the effect of root restriction on the overall plant size most convincingly.

Pruning the roots of a tree in the ground will result in a proportional amount of the canopy dying back. It is a procedure which is extremely physically demanding and will probably need to be done annually. This form of root restriction is unlikely to be useful for our purposes, and anyone who is prepared to spend a winter's day digging a trench a metre deep around a firm-rooted tree will probably have few problems with climbing a ladder at harvest time.

Restricting a plant to a container is far more likely to serve our needs. There is a wide range of fruit trees that will quite happily grow and fruit abundantly while growing in a pot. Care of container-grown plants is dealt with in detail in a later section, in Chapter 6. Here it will suffice to say that they require more routine maintenance than plants growing in the ground. It is necessary to be diligent about both feeding and watering. However, harvesting can be done from the ground, as can pruning. The usual principles of formative pruning and training apply to container-grown trees. Fruit trees that are suitable for growing in pots include small citrus trees such as cumquats and Meyer lemons or a larger variety on a dwarfing root stock. Quinces, figs and feijoas are also suitable as are the dwarf peaches and nectarines and, of course, apples on dwarfing rootstocks.

Another method of restricting root growth may be offered by the felted root control bags used in the production of advanced trees. These bags are used to grow advanced trees in the ground while containing the roots within the tufted fabric. They are currently being assessed to find out if it is possible to maintain certain fruit trees in the bags long term. It is too early to draw any firm conclusions; some results look promising while others have established that particularly vigorous root systems such as that of the mulberry will penetrate the root control bags in time.

Planting trees close together or even in the same hole is another way of restricting root growth, thereby limiting the final size of the tree. This rather extends the choice of 'smaller growing' plants available to us. By selecting the less vigorous varieties and planting them close to each other, the final size of the trees will be reduced. Two plants of the same species can be planted together in the same hole at the same time. For fruit varieties that require a cross-pollinator, a pollinating variety is the obvious choice for a near neighbour.

Training the canopy

Many of the fruit trees we commonly grow in the home garden can be trained to reach no more than two or three metres. To do so, it is necessary to commence training with the young trees at the time of planting. The trees can be grown as free standing specimens, or grown against some form of support. They can be trained into a smaller version of their natural shape, or coaxed into a stylised form such as a horizontal espalier or an oblique cordon. In either case, the tree must receive a rigorous education throughout its early years—young wood must be tied, unwanted growth removed!

The timing and severity of the formative action required will vary according to the desired result, but generally, the more formal the shape, the more the work that is required in both its development and its maintenance. Before taking on the task of tree training, a gardener should consider whether the work involved suits their individual temperament: an enthusiastic fair weather gardener may welcome the summer pruning involved in growing a cordon or an espalier, while those who wilt in the summer sun will wisely opt for a form where pruning can be postponed to the cooler months. Consider *your* needs before those of the tree.

Formative training

Large fruit trees are often grown with the thought that the larger the tree, the more fruit will be produced. In fact, this is not always the case and many commercial orchards are now finding that they obtain better yields by planting smaller-growing trees in larger numbers. Despite this, home gardeners will still often find themselves faced with pruning instructions that will produce a tree that is larger than is desirable. Fruit trees are surprisingly flexible on the matter of size—of far greater importance to the fruitfulness of a tree is the presence of the type of wood that will bear the fruit.

The formative training, that is, the pruning, tying and otherwise shaping, involved in training small-growing trees is essentially that used with a full-sized tree. The difference lies merely in the size of the 'framework' that is established and maintained. In both cases the training is concerned with producing a strong and healthy tree that carries a sufficient amount of productive wood. Fruit trees that carry their fruit on permanent fruiting spurs are developed so that the framework includes these spurs. Trees that fruit on last year's wood are developed so that some old growth is replaced each year; this new growth can ripen over the season and bear fruit the following year.

With dwarf trees or those with restricted roots, the tree will simply grow on a smaller scale and training will proceed accordingly. Where the training is to be the *means* of obtaining a small-growing tree, the height above the ground chosen to develop the main boughs will be higher than otherwise. The fundamentals of the training remain the same. Some important points to keep in mind when pruning or otherwise training a fruit tree are listed below:

—Light and air must be able to penetrate the canopy. Good fruiting requires that as much as possible of the canopy be exposed to the sun. Good air circulation is important in preventing disease.

—The tree must have a basic structure that is strong enough to support the ripened fruit. Sharp angles between the trunk and a main bough, or a bough and a lateral branch are weak—an angle significantly less than 45 degrees means the tree is in danger of splitting at the join. The angles will need to be widened (for example, by 'pegging down' a developing branch while the wood is still green) or the branch removed.

—Vertical branches are associated with growth while the more horizontally inclined are associated with fruiting. Some branches will need to be trained to grow more horizontally while others will need to be removed.

—Summer pruning will limit the tree's vegetative growth, whereas growth will be stimulated by pruning in winter.

—Removing an entire branch will redirect growth into the other parts of the tree. Removing part of a branch will cause growth from buds lower down that branch.

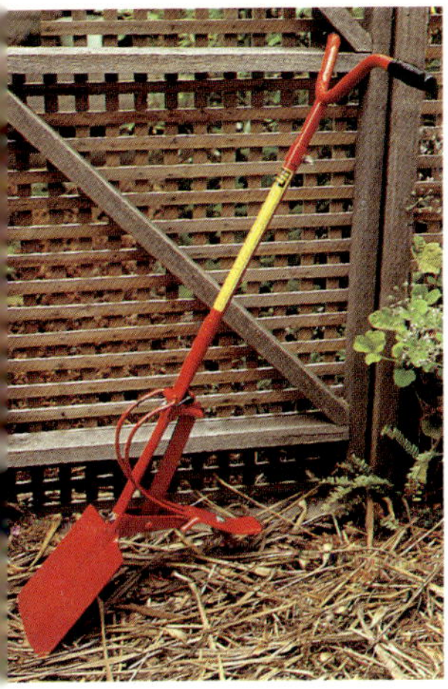

The Terex Auto Spade 37

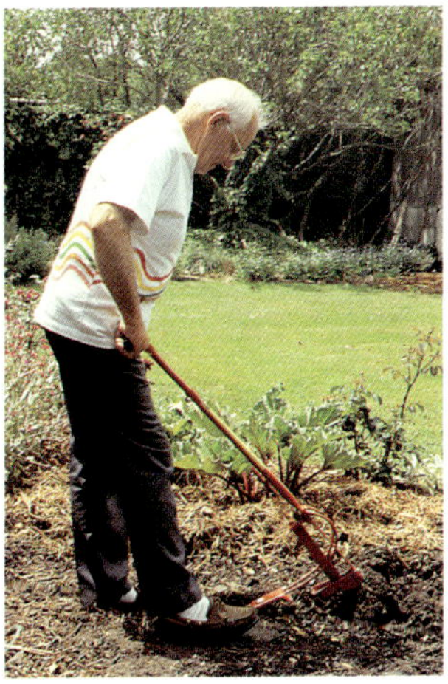

The Terex *in use* 38

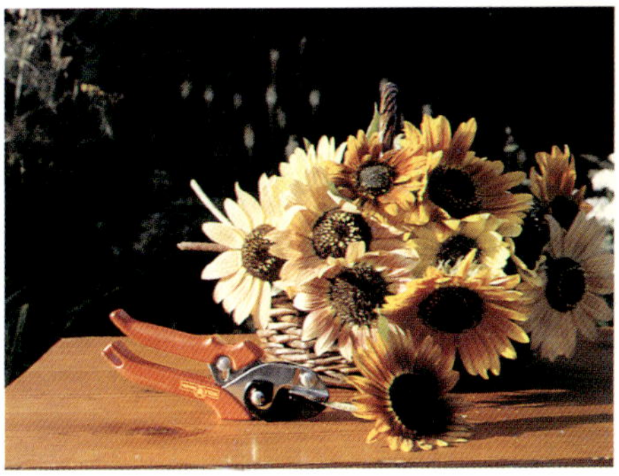

Wolf *'Cut-and-Hold' secateurs* 39

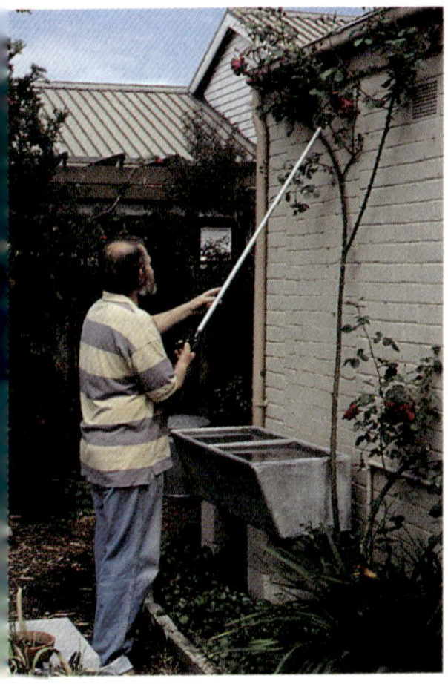

40

Long-handled 'Cut-and-Hold' pruners in use with a climbing rose

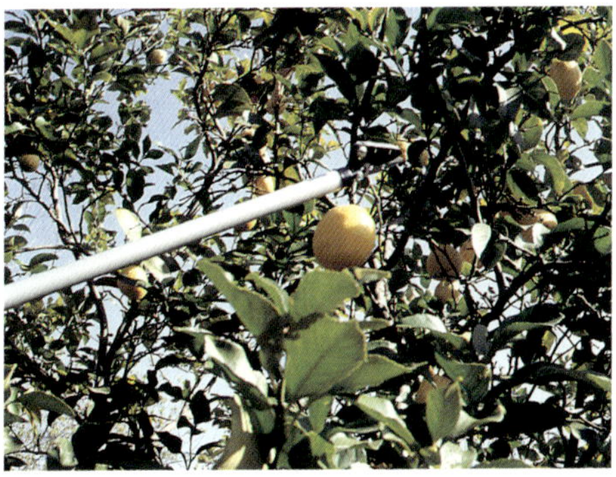

41

Kamaki *Cut-and-Hold pruners can be used to pick flowers or fruit*

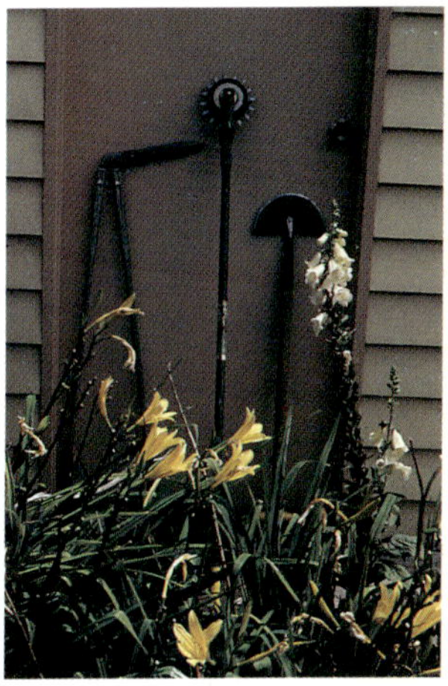

42

A selection of long-handled manual lawn edging tools

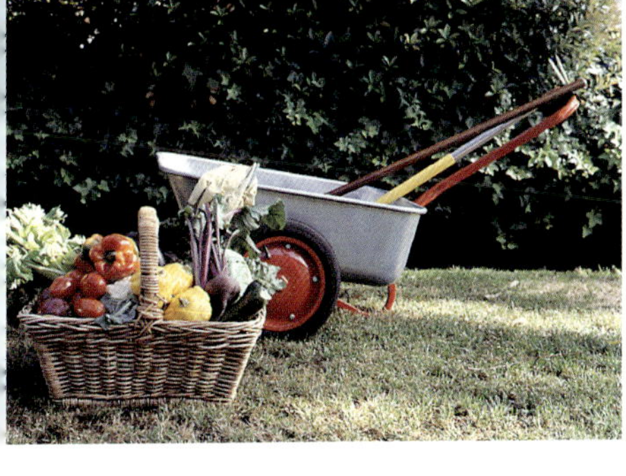

43

The easy to handle Daytek *twin-wheeled barrow*

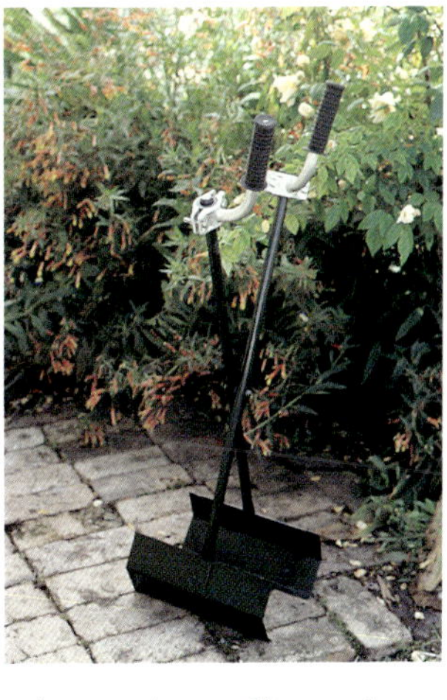

44

The Garden Gillie *with auxiliary handles for additional length*

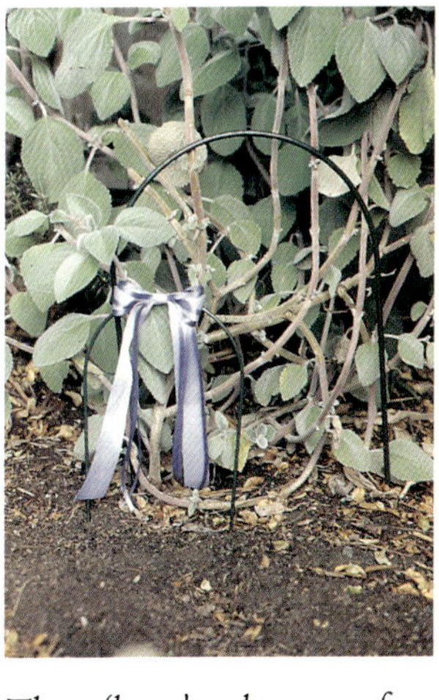

45

These 'hoop' stakes are safe, inconspicuous and effective

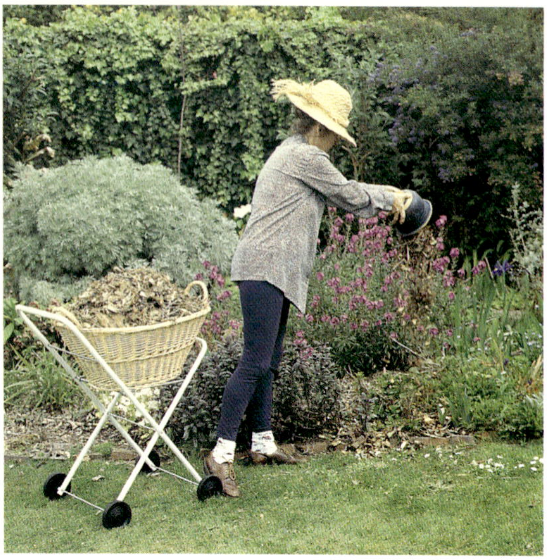

46

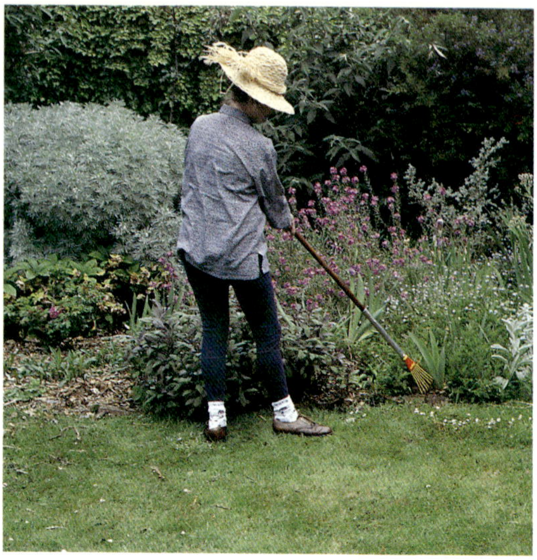

47

Above left: *Mulching — make it easy on your back — a laundry basket is a good way to transport mulch round the garden.*

Above right: *Mulch is easily spread using a small rake on a handle of a suitable length.*

Right: *A garden muncher — mulch as you go, the ideal situation.*

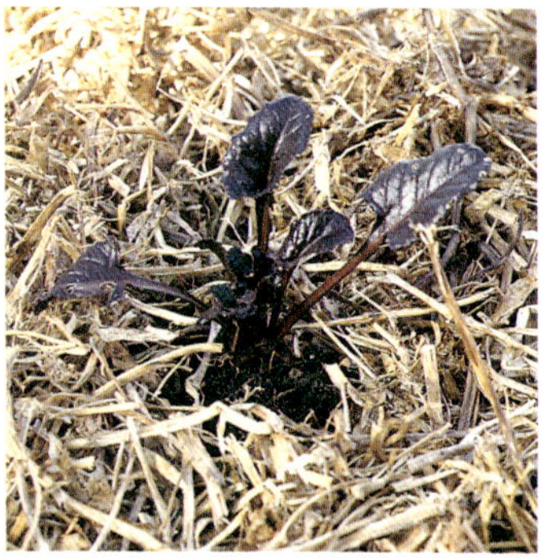

48

Seedlings are planted in a mound of compost within the layer of straw.

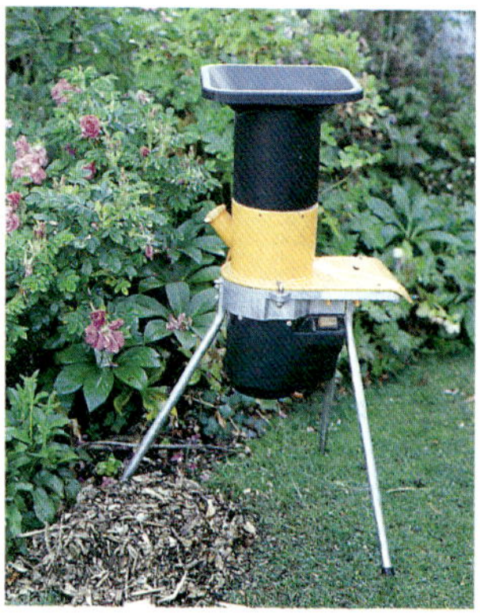

49

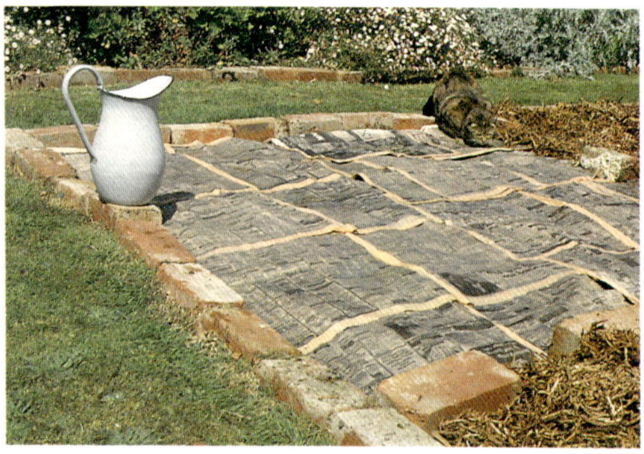

50

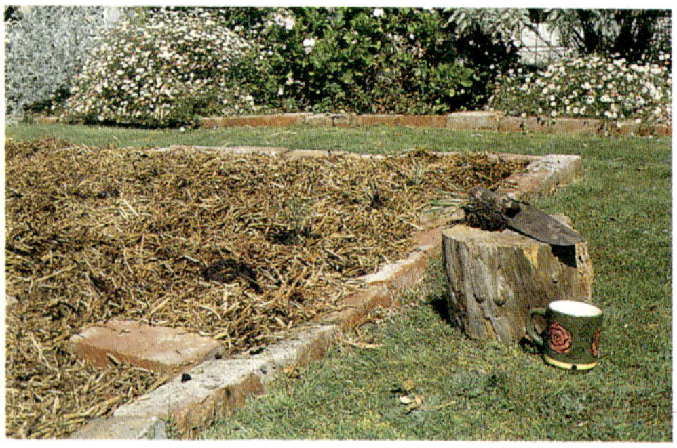

51

Top: *Newspaper laid as the bottom layer of a No-Dig garden. A thick layer of straw is laid on top of the newspaper*

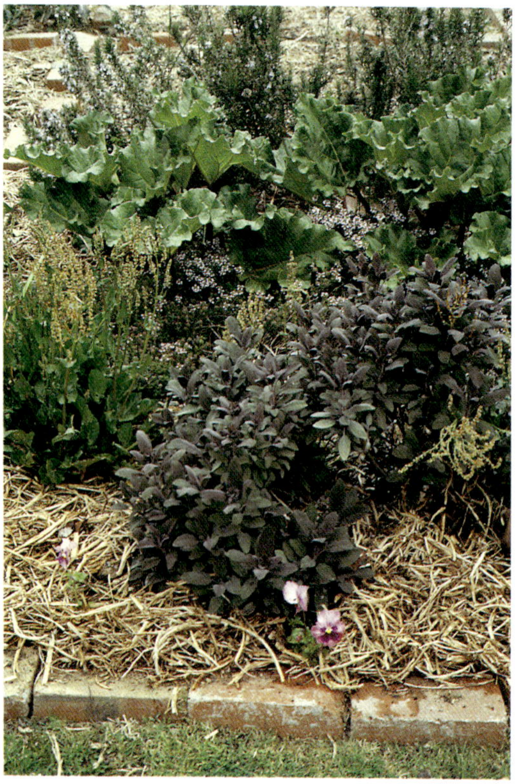

52

Perennials and annuals established and maintained in a No-Dig kitchen garden.

Of importance when training for easy access is that all the fruit-bearing parts of the tree must be easily and safely reached from the ground. In cases where fruit is borne on growth made the previous year this must be taken into account when developing the framework. If in doubt as to whether a tree bears its fruit on spurs or on last year's laterals, consult your local nursery or perhaps the wholesale nursery which supplies the trees to the local nursery. As a rule of thumb, apples and pears are spur-bearers although a few varieties, such as Golden Delicious, are lateral bearers. Stone fruit are usually lateral bearers, although apricots at maturity will carry a good deal of their fruit on spurs.

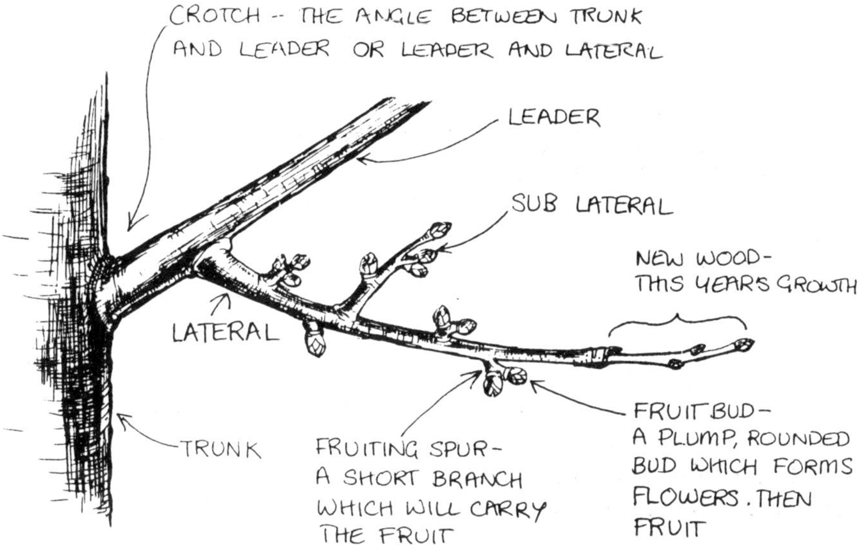

A pictorial glossary for fruit trees.

How to train a free-standing tree for easy reaching

The *Vase-* or *V-shaped* tree is the most suitable for a free-standing tree in the garden from our point of view. It can be used for all kinds of deciduous trees. This shape has a short trunk with three of four main branches that grow at an open angle to the trunk. These main branches are referred to as *leaders*. These leaders branch again, giving perhaps six or eight branches in the framework. Be aware that once growth becomes woody it does not grow in length anymore. Thus a branch arising 20 cm (8″) above the ground from a two-year-old woody trunk will remain at 20 cm height throughout its life.

To develop a low-growing vase-shaped tree, the following procedure should be followed: Fruit trees are usually supplied to the nurseries at the end of their second year. By then, some branching should have been developed. Select a young tree that has three or four branches arising from the trunk at around 30 cm (1′) from the ground. Trim these selected branches back to 30 cm; remove any other branches at the trunk. Cut the central stem back to 60 cm (2′). This will redirect growth back into your chosen leaders. Branch angles can be opened up and branches made to grow more horizontally by the use of wooden spreaders or by tying them down to a peg in the ground.

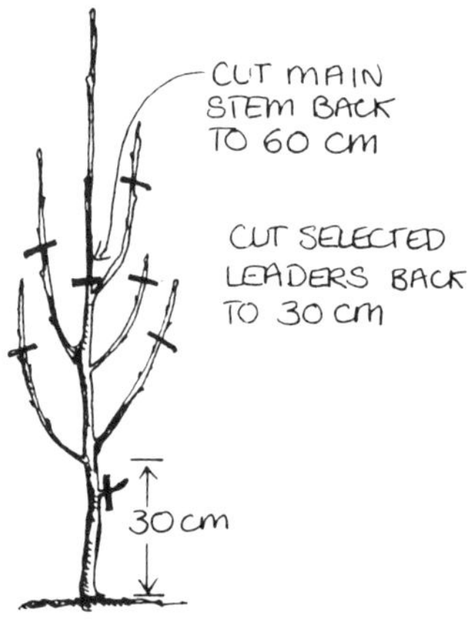

V-shaped tree-to-be at planting.

At the end of the first year of growth, the leaders should have branched. Select two or perhaps three branches from each leader. If unsure of where to cut, follow each branch through, see where it arises, see if it grows vertically upwards, or at more of an angle. See what contribution it will make to the framework—is the inside angle wide enough to ensure the join is strong, will the tree have a sound shape after including it? Chances are that your tree will not look like the one in the pruning book, but with a little commonsense and some careful observation, a pleasing and fruitful small tree will eventuate. It may well be necessary to prop the low-growing branches up when they are carrying fruit.

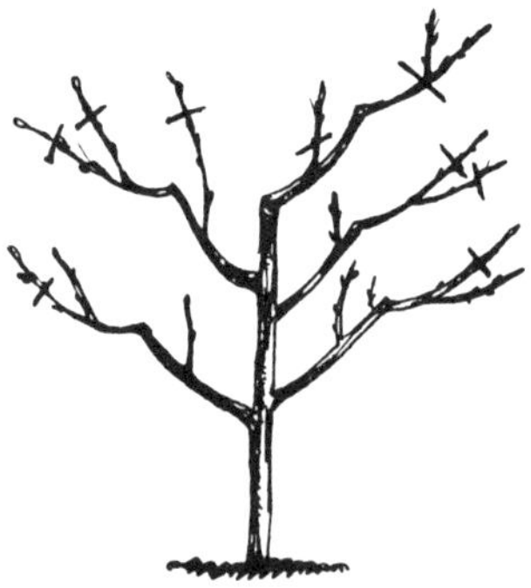

V-shaped tree after Year I.

In the following years the tree is pruned back to the basic structure which has been established during these early years. This is most conveniently done in winter when the bare branches make it easy to see what is happening. However, over-vigorous growth is best cut back in summer rather than winter to prevent even stronger growth resulting.

When pruning, dead and diseased wood should first be removed, as should any branches which cross or grow in towards the centre of the tree. In the case of spur-bearing varieties, retain all leaders that have fruited well. Cut back laterals that have grown beyond the leaders. As spurs age they become less fruitful and it may prove necessary to include suitable new wood in the framework to develop for future spur replacement. Any of the selected branches (of your framework) that have grown vigorously should be cut back by at least one-third, more if you think it is necessary for ease of access. Remove all unwanted growth.

How to train a supported tree that can be easily reached

Training trees against some form of support offers several advantages to the gardener. Firstly, the tree grows in only two dimensions and so takes up considerably less space. Because the branches are tied to assume a more horizontal position they can be made more fruitful. Although it is unreasonable to expect a tree growing in only two dimensions to produce as much fruit as if it were free-standing, because all parts of the tree are exposed to the sun, yields can be surprisingly high.

It may be possible to take advantage of a sunny wall for early ripening, or for shelter from prevailing winds. If a wall is not available as support, then a stout wire or lattice on posts can be used. For those who are really keen, a fruiting hedge can be developed by training a row of fruit trees to grow formally entwined with one another.

The regular geometric shapes that are traditionally used for supported trees are highly decorative and can be used to great advantage as either a backdrop or a feature. Add to this the accessibility of a tree trained low in two dimensions and it would seem to offer all that could be wished for. The drawback lies in the amount of work involved in shaping and maintaining these stylised forms. The challenge in training a tree in two dimensions lies in tying and pruning at the right time. Young wood must be bent and secured before it has hardened; summer pruning must be done each year at the end of the main growth season. These tasks must be done with great punctuality or form will be sacrificed!

Espaliered forms

An espalier is a vertically planted tree or shrub that is trained against a support. The branches can be trained as horizontal 'arms' or in more elaborate 'candelabra' forms. These shapes are better suited to spur-bearing trees such as apple or pear. Trees can also be trained into a fan-shaped espalier. This shape is better suited to the lateral-bearing stone fruits such as peach and cherry. Free-form espaliers may take a gardener's fancy, and so long as the tree's needs are being met, then why not?! Judicious selection of smaller varieties or even dwarf trees is advisable for all espaliers.

Although customarily used for deciduous fruit trees, espalier can be used just as effectively for evergreens—A small citrus tree could be used to give an espalier that is useful as well as attractive. Some beautiful espaliers have been produced using evergreen ornamentals such as Sasanqua camellias and *Garrya elliptica* (Necklace Bush).

How to train a horizontal espalier Select a young tree with three strong buds about 30 cm (1′) from the ground. Cut the stem back to just above the buds at planting, with the buds arranged as shown.

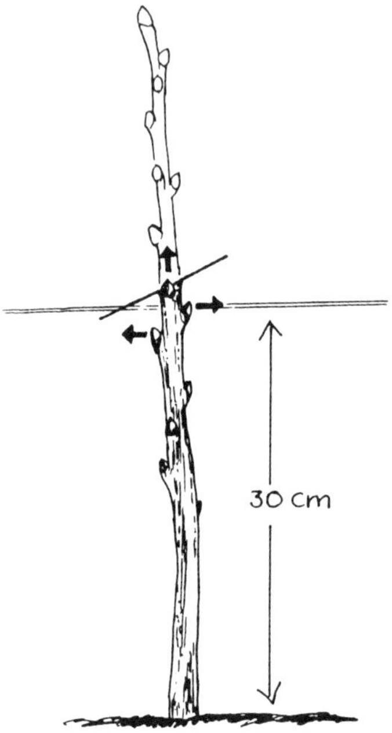

An espalier-to-be at planting.

In the first summer, when the buds have grown into branches of around 50 cm (1′8″), secure them to stakes. Fasten the stakes to horizontal wires attached to a support and arranged in tiers starting at around 30 cm (1′) above the ground, and with 40–60 cm (1′4″–2′) between them in the vertical direction. The central shoot is trained to grow vertically. The two side shoots are initially tied at an angle of 45 degrees.

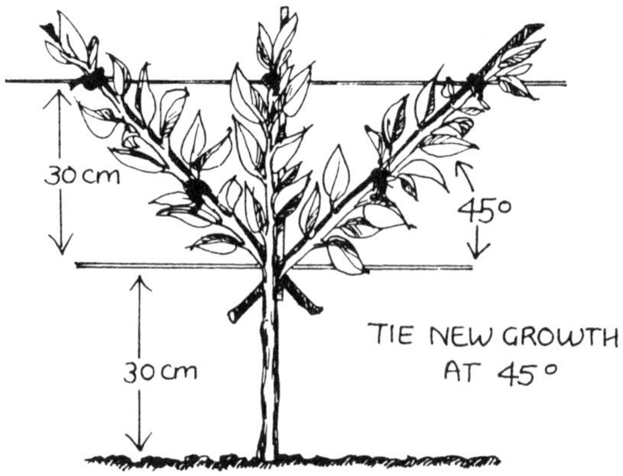

Training in the first summer.

By the end of the first year the two side shoots should have grown sufficiently to tie horizontally along the lowest wire. Two buds arising near the second tier can then be tied to the stakes and fastened at 45 degrees. At the end of the season they too should be long enough to tie horizontally along the next tier. This is repeated yearly until the desired number of tiers is obtained.

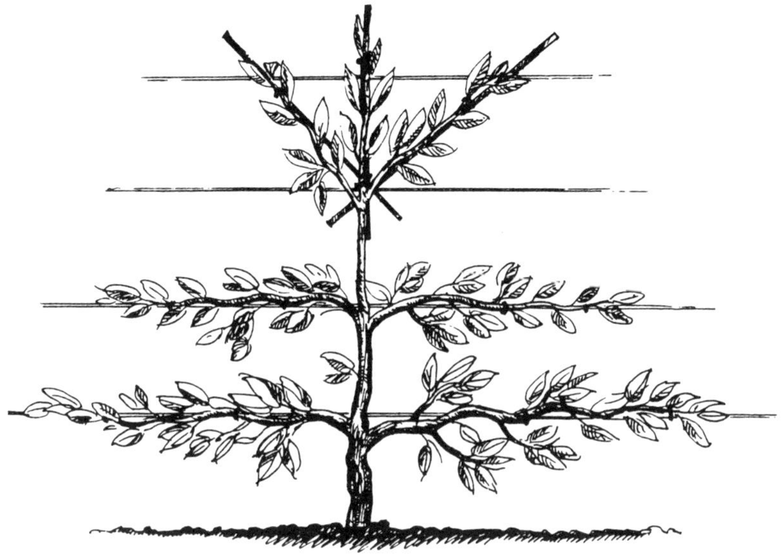

Training after the first year.

Each summer, remove all growth from the central stem (except for that needed for the next horizontal layer during establishment, or for spur renewal in the mature tree). Remove any strong vertical shoots growing along the horizontally trained branches, while any shoots that have made moderate growth should be cut back to three or four buds.

How to train a fan-shaped espalier Fan-shaped espaliers are suitable for lateral bearing fruit trees. There are two styles of fan-shaped espalier. The more formal style is trained in a manner very similar to the horizontal espalier. It features a central trunk with pairs of branches coming off it, in this case trained at 70 degrees to the inside angle with the trunk (the 'head-and-shoulders' angle, not the 'armpit').

Two styles of fan-shaped espalier.

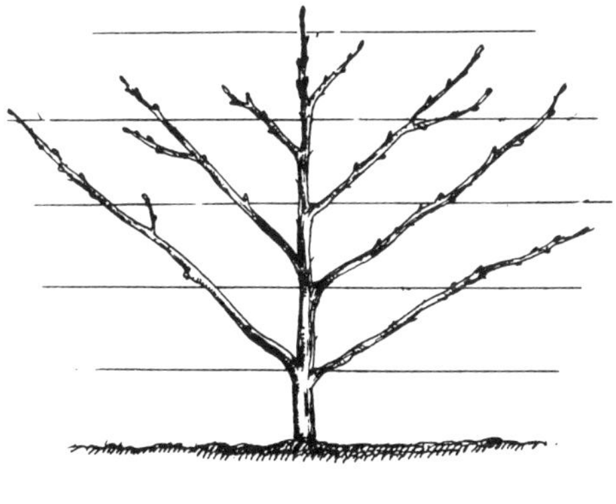

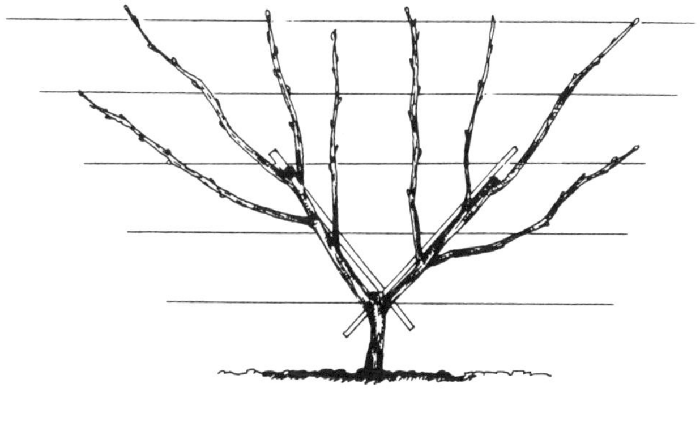

A more free-form style of fan is developed by training two shoots at 45 degrees. The central stem is removed. Each side shoot is allowed to branch into two each season, and these shoots are tied into the support.

Cordons The name 'cordon' is of French origin and means 'rope' or 'cord'. A tree cordon is planted at an angle, and growth confined to the single trunk and very short laterals. The oblique planting considerably reduces the size and the vigour of the tree, but even so, dwarf trees are recommended. Summer pruning must be carried out to remove unwanted growth. It is suitable only for spur-bearers.

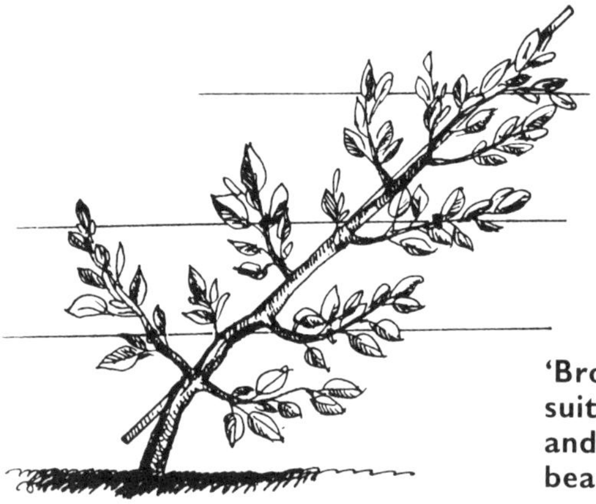

'English Cordon'—suitable only for spur-bearers.

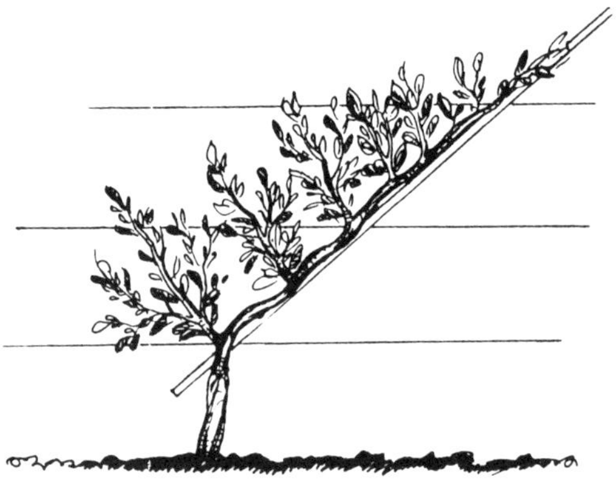

'Broad Cordon'—suitable for spur- and lateral-bearers.

A Spot of Science

Plant growth requirements

For a plant to grow to its full potential all of its needs must be met. Plant growth is affected by temperature, by the level of light and the availability of water, carbon dioxide and oxygen as well as a number of nutrients it must obtain from the soil. An adequate level of all these requirements must be supplied for a plant to grow well. But enough is as good as a feast—in some cases, supplying a plant with too much of these can actually lead to a decrease in the growth rate.

The optimum level for each of these factors will vary from plant to plant and again is the result of a plant having adapted to its native environment. For example, a plant grows best over its native range of temperature—growth will increase as the temperature rises within this range but will drop off towards the extremes. Some plants have a particular temperature requirement for a specific part of their life cycle. An example of this is the winter dormancy that some plants require in order to induce flowering.

While flowers and fruit are often the reason for us including a plant in our gardens, they are involved only in the sexual reproduction of the plant and in fact are not essential for 'everyday' plant functions. They do not help a plant to adapt to a particular environment but often themselves have very specific requirements for their development. The amount of light that a plant receives as well as the length of the days are factors that commonly infuence flowering.

All plants need to lose a certain amount of water by evaporation through tiny pores on the surface of their leaves. Some plants have adapted to a particular native environment by developing structures to regulate the rate of this evaporation; for example, some dry climate plants have a thick, waxy coating on their leaves to cut down evaporation, while others conserve their moisture by reducing the number of pores on the leaf surface.

An often overlooked requirement for good plant growth is oxygen. Most plants get their oxygen from the air that is held in the soil. A soil that is waterlogged will contain no air and plants can drown in these conditions just as surely as can their human counterparts. Only a few plants that are normally found growing with their feet in water are able to use the oxygen produced by their leaves in photosynthesis.

A little soil science

A good, well managed soil is essential for the well-being of the plants. The soil is a vibrant, dynamic amalgum of many varied substances and our horticultural success depends upon its health. The biological properties of the soil are of immense importance; the presence of soil dwelling organisms, both microscopic and those that can be seen with the naked eye, are vital to the soundness of a soil. In addition to these living creatures, the soil is made up of three main components.

The first of these is the MINERAL PARTICLES. These particles are formed from weathered rock; the size of the particles determines the basic soil type or texture. Large particles, that is, for a soil, are found in sandy soils, while the particles of a clay soil are fine. Pure loam has particles of an intermediate size, while clay loams and sandy loams have particles of a size that lie in between the main types. The coarse particles of a sand allow water to penetrate rapidly, but relatively little is retained. Nutrients are easily leached, that is, washed out, from sandy soils. Water will penetrate a clay soil less rapidly but more of it is retained. Clay also retains nutrients well. The other soil types have properties that lie between the two extremes.

The second soil component is ORGANIC MATTER. This comes from a number of sources. Some come from the plant material that has fallen on the soil surface, such as fallen leaves and spent annuals. Manure is deposited by passing animals. Further organic matter comes from within the soil; dying roots as well as secretions and excretions of soil dwellers all make a contribution. Organic matter releases nutrients gradually to the plants in a form that they can utilise. Organic matter will improve water penetration in a clay soil and increase water retention in a sandy one. It brings about many positive changes to the chemical nature, the biological activity and the structure of the soil.

The final and frequently overlooked soil component is the HOLES. These spaces between the particles, more correctly termed 'pores', have a huge influence on the behaviour of a soil. In fact, some soil scientists would have it that the particles are only important because of the gaps between them!

Large pores allow rapid water penetration, good aeration and are easily penetrated by growing roots. However, they do not retain water well and allow leaching of valuable nutrients; large pores are to be found between the large particles of sandy soils. Small pores, on the other hand, do not allow the water to infiltrate so rapidly but will retain much more of it. These small pores, found in clay soils, are more likely to become waterlogged and to impede root growth. A mixture of both large and small pores will provide good water retention, good aeration and good water infiltration.

Soil structure

These individual components are drawn together to form a structured soil by the action of soil-dwelling organisms. Mineral particles and organic matter are bound into 'crumbs' by the sticky secretions of feeding microbes. Both fungi and bacteria produce strands and slimes that glue the particles together into larger aggregates. Earthworms and other small soil animals produce a network of continuous tunnels. Plant roots growing through the soil will eventually die and decay, further adding to the tunnelling. The continuity of the spaces is important as it aids the passage of both water and air and also provides the best conditions for root growth and other biological activity. Over time, and with an adequate supply of organic matter, the efforts of the soil dwellers produce the desired continuity and variation in pore size. Over-cultivation and compaction are two of the many ways to destroy a soil structure that will have taken years to create.

A little soil chemistry

The mineral particles in the soil are made up of a large number of different elements. These elements are present in the parent rock in forms which are of little nutritional value to most plants or animals. These parent rocks have been weathered by the wind and the rain for millions of years. They have been acted upon by countless generations of soil microbes that have converted the minerals to soluble organic compounds; these can then be utilised by the plants.

All mineral nutrients must be taken up from the soil in the correct form and dissolved in water. The plant needs to obtain certain nutrients from the soil in relatively large amounts. These major elements are nitrogen, phosphorus, potassium, calcium and magnesium. Other elements are needed in smaller amounts. These, the trace elements, are iron, manganese, copper, zinc, boron and molybdenum. Chloride may also be needed.

'pH' is a measure of acidity and alkalinity. A pH value of around 7 is neutral. A pH value above 7 is alkaline; below 7 is acidic. Many living organisms have only a small range of pH over which they can live and this is so of soil organisms. These micro-organisms are important not just for the effect they have on the soil structure. In many cases, plants are dependent on particular microbes to make certain essential nutrients available for their use. And indeed the mere presence of non-harmful co-dwelling micro-organisms, even if of no direct benefit, is important in controlling disease-causing microbes simply by competing with them for resources.

While most plants can grow over a relatively large pH range, they too have their limits. Furthermore, pH affects the availability of nutrients to the plants. Most of these elements are at their most available at a neutral pH, usually between 6.5–7.00.

A number of things can affect the pH of the soil and hence plant growth. The presence of organic matter has a buffering effect and will prevent any large changes in pH in most conditions. Organic matter is important for its ability to maintain soil pH as well as for its nutrient value and its contribution to soil structure.

5
Garden Layout

A GARDEN IS A PLACE WE GO TO BE MOST OURSELVES; THERE WE CAN TOUCH nature, feel the passing of the seasons; there we can just let ourselves 'be'. It is a place that evokes a strong emotional response in us, where the whole is so much more than the sum of the individual parts. It is the spirit of a garden in which the magic resides, not the bricks and mortar, the cunning design or beautiful plants, however fine these may be.

However, a garden is not only a set of 'intangibles'; it is also a physical place. As such, a garden will be worked in, lived in, moved through, sat in and looked upon, and the quality of this physical environment will clearly affect us. As we grow older, our safety and comfort within the garden become important considerations. Shelter and shade should be provided; permanent features such as paths, patios, steps and seating should be designed and constructed with due attention to convenience and protection as well as to appearance—there should be no slippery paths, no precipitous dips, no treacherous steps or perpendicular plunges. Utility areas should be easily and conveniently reached, plants restrained in areas where they could pose some risk. A well designed garden will allow easy access throughout, with unexpected delights but no hidden dangers. It will be workable, comfortable, useful and beautiful, all according to the needs and desires of the individual gardener.

The majority of us will remain in our family homes on retiring, but a growing number are now moving house on or around the time of retirement, in search of a more congenial climate, a better life-style or a more easily maintained home. Both situations present us with challenges and opportunities in the garden. Those who stay in their original homes may find commonsense dictating that they modify some of the features they have loved and lived with for years or even decades; this is not always an easy thing to do. Those who move may well have to start from scratch in the garden, with all the headaches and hassles that this can involve. In either case, timely attention to the design and construction of the 'built' garden elements can be crucial to making a smooth transition into gardening in our later years.

Hard landscape is the term given to these built, non-living elements of a garden, such as paving, pergolas, water features and retaining walls. The hard landscaping influences the way we utilise the garden, and in some cases actually determines how a particular area will be used. For example, paths will be walked along to get from one part of the garden to the next, steps will be used to reach different levels within the garden, while paved seating areas will be used to sit and socialise in. At least, this will be the case if they are well placed and well constructed. Hard landscaping can be used to create microclimates within the garden that will extend the range of plants that can be grown; it can be used, too, to buffer the human inhabitants of the garden from both the physical and emotional assaults of the outer world.

As well as affecting its functional aspects, the hard landscape will contribute to the beauty of a garden. In addition to providing a setting for the plants—the real business of a garden for most people—the hard elements can carry a garden through the lean times when there may be little seasonal interest in the vegetation. These built features can also have a profound effect on the atmosphere of a garden, on the way a garden *feels*. Changes in level, enclosures, subdivisions, a partially concealed view not only make an aesthetic contribution but also evoke in us primordial emotional responses which hark back to times early in our evolution. Then we needed to 'read' the landscape at a glance in terms of concealment, shelter, escape routes, exposure to predators. We will still do this, though largely at the subconscious level, and experience a consequent emotional response. Added to these responses will be a lifetime of associations with different land forms and features. We bring to these also a sense of scale and proportion and a set of responses that develop as a result of our personal preferences and our particular physical and cultural environments.

However, our home environments are far from being safe havens—An analysis of accidents involving older people, both in Australia and the USA, has revealed that around half of all falls (the largest category of accidents involving the elderly, and a major cause of death and disability in this group) occur at home. It appears that we are at risk out of doors in transition areas, that is, areas where some change occurs, such as going from the dark into the bright light, on steps, or where there is a change in surfacing materials. It would seem that we need to pay a little more attention to safety in these areas than we have done in the past.

For all these reasons, the built elements warrant our full attention in the initial stages of designing or redesigning the garden. The first step is to list all the things that we require from a garden. Features such as a paved eating area, a pond, a screened area for the clothes line, a path to the garden shed may appear on the list. Considerations such as privacy, shielding from noise or a sense of spaciousness should also be listed. List each and every thing that your heart desires—they may not all be possible within the constraints of space and budget, but at least by listing them we will be better able to sort out priorities and see just what we can achieve.

Hard Surfaces

It is over hard surfaces that we will usually be moving when we pass through these high-risk transition areas; both the design and the materials used will affect how safe a surface is. That it should also be properly constructed goes without saying—a badly laid surface will soon become cracked and uneven and may end up being more difficult and hazardous than the original, unpaved state.

A hard surface will act as a heatbank, soaking up the warmth during the day, then releasing it later as the ambient temperature drops. This is something we most of us welcome in the milder months; however, in summertime this asset can turn into a liability as patios and paths throw the heat back at us as the sun goes down. We need to consider carefully where we site our paving, and provide shade or water for cooling where we wish to avoid a heat trap.

Drainage

Hard surfaces will collect a surprising amount of water, thus it is essential that the surface water drain away. There are two main reasons for this. Firstly, if the paved area is to be used in all weathers it must not have water lying on its surface. Secondly, damp conditions will encourage the growth of moss and algae; this will render even the most slip-resistant of surfaces perilous in the extreme. Paving must always have a slight slope to allow the water to run off. The water from smaller surfaces such as paths and steps can usually be safely run off onto the adjoining ground, but with larger areas of paving such as patios and terraces the water should run off into a drainage pit set towards a corner of the paving. The grills of the pits can be highly decorative, many beautiful wrought iron designs are available. Make sure that the openings of the grill are not of a width that could catch walking sticks or aids—or stiletto heels. The drainage pit will connect with the stormwater drainage system. Water can sometimes be allowed to drain onto an adjoining garden bed instead; this will depend on factors such as how well the bed itself drains, the nature of the planting and whether or not it will create a problem with soil erosion. Water must *never*, under any circumstances, drain towards the house. A fall of 1:60 is the standard slope for a paved area; this drop should be included from the start of the design process.

Choice of materials

Paving should look attractive as well as being functional; both aspects deserve due consideration. However, not all the materials commonly used for paving are safe in outdoor areas and only materials that have enough slip resistance when wet should be considered. Similarly, rough surfaces such as gravels or highly textured surfaces should be avoided. These are difficult to negotiate for anyone with a mobility problem, so increasing the likelihood of a fall, and if an older person were to trip on this surface, the risk of serious abrasions to a thinned elderly skin (see Chapter 1) is high. Loose stones can also be inadvertently carried over onto smooth surfaces; because they are easily overlooked and unexpected, they can prove extremely hazardous in these circumstances.

Timber, terrazo, as well as some natural stones, smooth finished concrete and non slip-resistant ceramic products are unsuitable. However, it may be possible to improve the grip of some existing surfaces. Procedures such as sand blasting, acid etching and some newly developed proprietory treatments can increase slip resistance on some surfaces. Consult *Standards Australia*, document AS 1428–1, for suitable treatments for different surfaces; the engineering department of your local council will have a copy of this document.

There is still little guidance available to the public on commercially available 'do it yourself' products and unfortunately some treatments are only effective in the short term. If you would like to use them on your existing surfaces, you are best to contact your State Independent Living Centre, who may be able to help you with information on the matter. Where a suitable treatment cannot be found, non-slip mats are an option for high usage areas.

If all that sounds too restrictive, fear not, there are many old garden favourites that can safely be used. Slip-resistant tiles and brick pavers, and natural stone with a rough finish are suitable; so too are textured concretes.

Brick pavers

All pavers that are sold as such must comply with the Australian Standard on slip resistance. Slip resistance has been expressed for years by the intriguingly titled 'British Pendulum Number' (BPN). As of October 1993, this has been replaced by the 'Coefficient of Friction' (COF), though some manufacturers still use the old term in their literature. A minimum Coefficient of Friction of 0.4 is required for pavers; this corresponds to a BPN of 40. Pavers will have a BPN that lies in the range of 40 to 80, but ideally, for older people, pavers with a BPN of between 55 to 75 (COF of 0.55–0.75) should be used.

The slip resistance of a paver is considered to be 'technical information' and one sometimes has to press the retailers to obtain the actual figure. Bricks that are sold as building bricks are not tested for slip resistance. Some may seem to promise a non-slip surface, but appearances can be deceptive—they are always an unknown quantity. Paving bricks are also different in size to building bricks and are much easier to lay in patterns where the bricks are laid at 90° to one another, such as basket weave and herringbone.

'Old reds'—recycled red building bricks—are extremely popular for garden paving. The general opinion is that they provide a reasonable, slip-resistant surface. However, this is only anecdotal evidence and not hard fact. Over time the brick will have developed micro-fissures in which moss and algae will flourish and regular maintenance may be necessary to keep the surface safe. The edges of the bricks will be broken and uneven to some extent, and so they should be groated using either a wet groat or mortar, whatever is appropriate for the sub-base used.

The choice of colour from amongst suitably low-slip pavers, happily, is large; however, safety considerations rule out using some tones. Our vision deteriorates as we age, in many cases quite seriously, and we should avoid colours which further reduce our visual perception (see Chapter 1). Light tones reflect light, thereby adding to the glare on bright days, and so should not be used, particularly by those who already have some loss of central field vision. Dark colours can be difficult to perceive, and can be particularly deceptive when used around changes in level and in shady places. Mid-tones are often the most successful in the garden in any case, so this restriction will probably not prove problematic. If you do feel the need to use either very dark or very light pavers, perhaps because you want to tie the paving in to some similarly toned permanent feature, use this 'difficult' colour in small amounts. Different colours can be successfully used in paving patterns, but refrain from using strongly contrasting colours as this can 'bewilder' our vision; busy, complicated patterns should be avoided for the same reason.

It may be helpful to define boundaries by using a row of lighter bricks at the edges. If a 'tactile' edging is more appropriate, this can be obtained by using a row of bricks turned on their sides so that they sit 'proud' above the paving, or by using purpose-made 'Dot-Dash' edging bricks that are designed to provide tactile clues to the visually impaired and are available from the larger brick manufacturers.

There are many different traditional patterns that brick pavers can be laid in. There are no rights and wrongs when selecting patterns, but if you are unsure of what would best please you in your garden, then use the following guidelines:

—Paving patterns (and colours) should not be at odds with the house and other permanent features.

—Patterns that are strongly 'directional' such as Stretcher Bond or 90° Herringbone work will in formal, geometric gardens.

—Basketweave and Circular brickwork marry happily with informal, cottage-style gardens. (45° Herringbone looks well with both formal and informal gardens.)

Laying brick paving It is essential that paving is properly laid. Badly laid paving will eventually break up, becoming both ugly and dangerous in the process. If you are laying the paving yourself, there are many books available that give clear step-by-step instructions on paving. Many of the larger paving manufacturers have 'how to' leaflets that cover paving methods suitable for most sites. If you are paying someone to do it, make sure you choose a reputable contractor to carry out the work. In either case, make sure that all the following points are considered:

1. Install subsurface drainage if your intended site does not drain adequately.
2. Excavate to the required depth, allowing sufficient depth for sub-base, sand or mortar bed and pavers. Never pave over topsoil; the organic content of the topsoil will cause too much movement as it shrinks and expands. Make sure the topsoil is saved for use in the garden—if you can think of no immediate use for it, use it to layer your compost heap as it builds up. Excavate to a fall of 1:60, draining away from any building. This fall will be carried right through to the final paving surface—make sure that it is correct at all levels. A drainage pit should be used for all large areas of paving; this pit must itself drain into the stormwater drainage system and needs to be connected before the paving is laid. Make sure the grill of the drainage pit does not have openings that are large enough (2 cm/0.8″) to catch a walking stick.
3. The thickness of the sub-base and the material used should be appropriate to the situation; both the amount of 'movement' expected of the soil *and* the amount of traffic the area will carry will need to be considered. Crushed rock will be adequate as a sub-base for stable to moderately stable soils, while unstable soils or an area that will carry vehicles will require a reinforced concrete slab as a sub-base. The pavers will then be laid on a bed of sand over a crushed rock base, while a mortar bed is used over a concrete slab. If unsure how

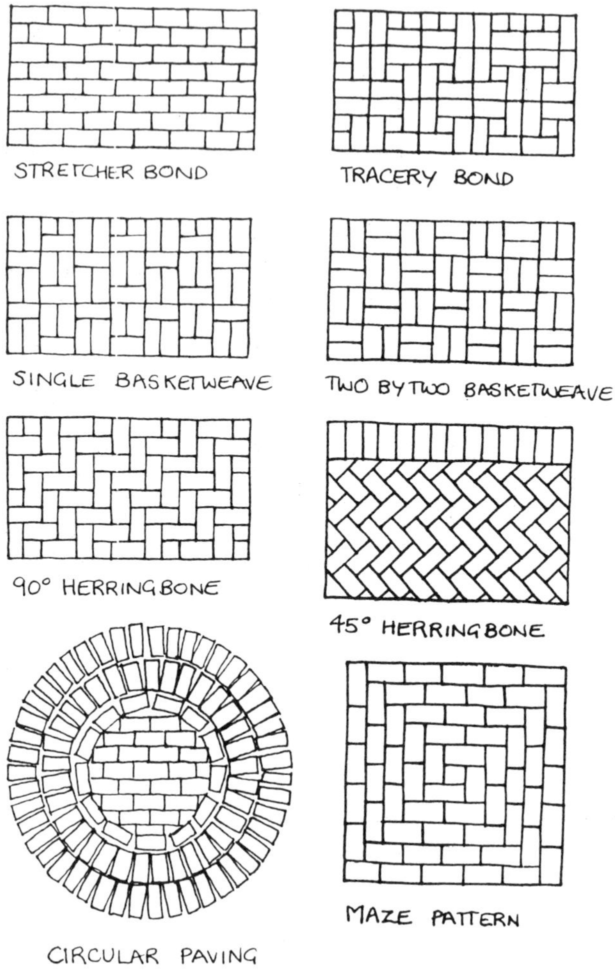

Some traditional paving patterns.

stable the soil in your area is, contact the Surveyors Department of your local shire or council.

4. Where crushed rock and sand have been used for the sub-base and the bed, then a vibrator should be used to compact the layers. These can be hired from tool-hire firms.
5. Pavers set on a mortar base should be groated (that is, the gaps between the bricks filled in) with mortar; when set on sand, use sand as the groat. A dry mixture of cement and sand—50/50—can be used to fill the gaps, then hosed down. This will harden on drying, but there is little control over the strength achieved and the groat may 'fail'. A disadvantage of using sand as your groat is that seeds will readily germinate in the sand, thus it lends itself to weed growth.
6. Edge restraints are essential—the free edges of the paving must be restrained by concrete haunching or some other form of fixed curbing. Failure to restrain the edges will lead to the paving breaking up, crumbling first at the unrestrained boundaries.

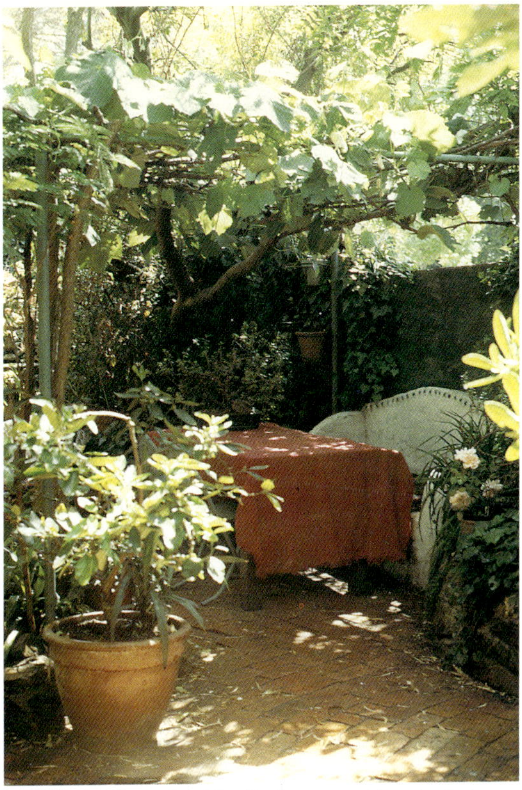

53

A pergola planted with climbers provides shade in two or three years. Here an out-door dining area is shaded by a grape vine.

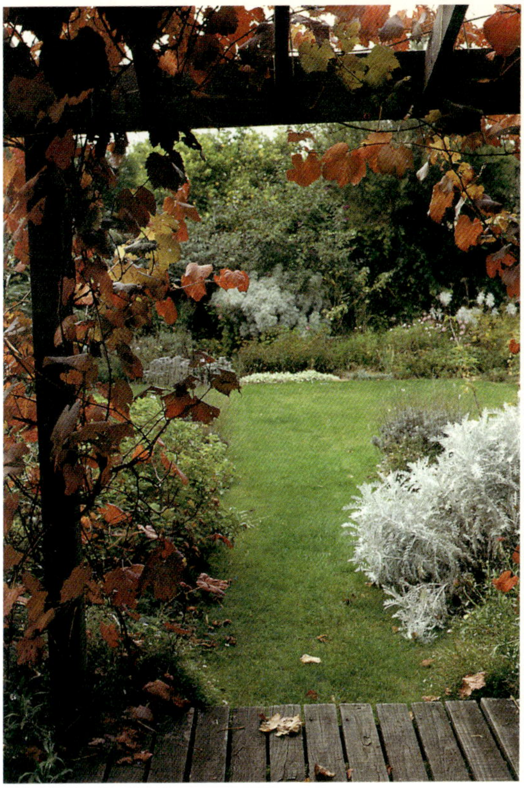

54

This vine-clad pergola shades the back of the house in summer and provides seasonal interest to this view from the kitchen.

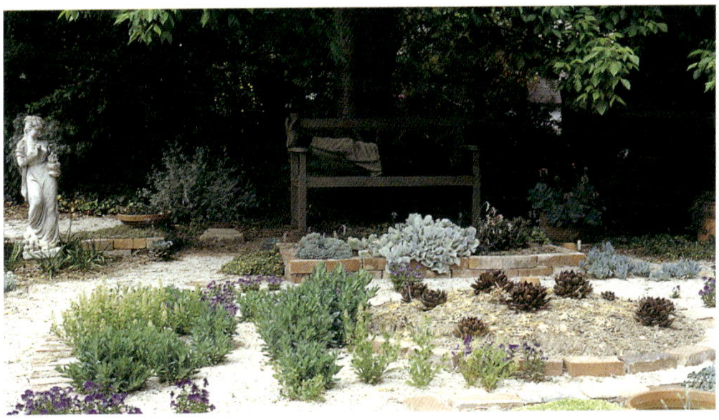

The deep shade of a mature tree for shade-loving gardeners. (Barbara Maund) 55

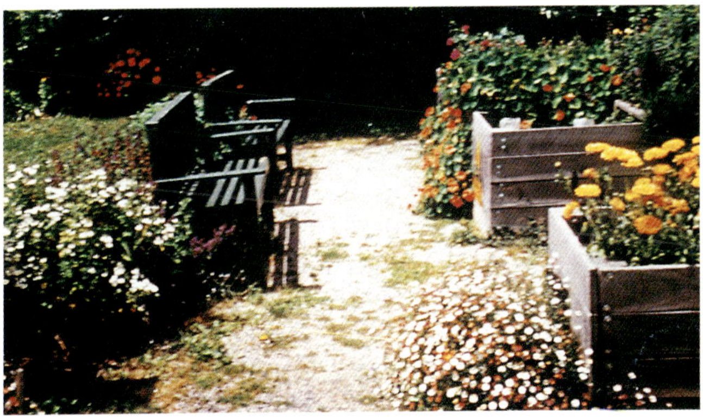

Raised garden beds planted with graceful trailing plants. 56

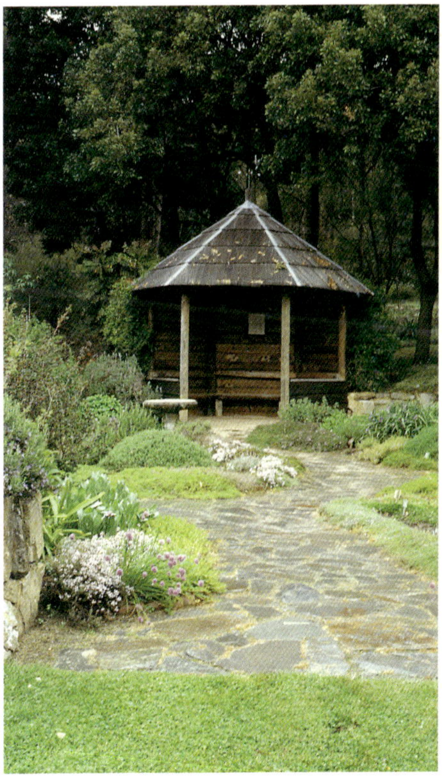

A Gazebo provides instant shade for the gardener. (Garden of St Erth) 57

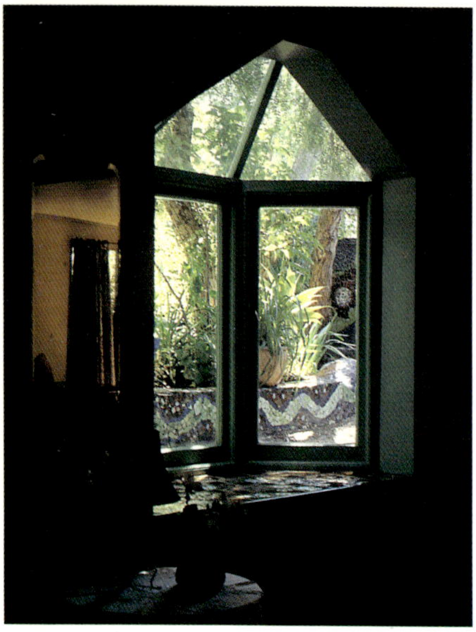

58

Prioritise those areas in the garden that give the most pleasure—a view from a window can be most important. (Margot Knox's Mosaic Garden)

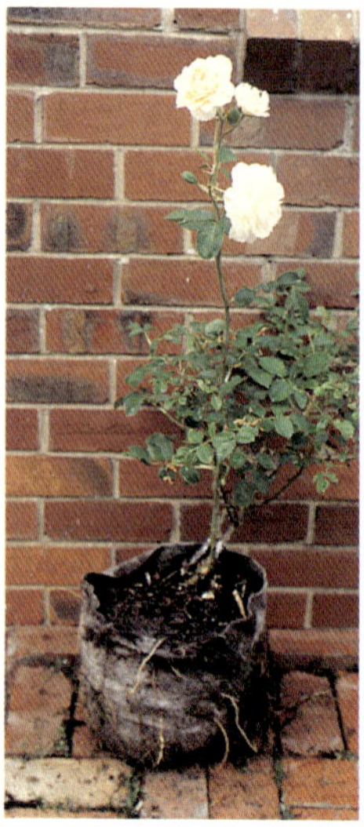

59

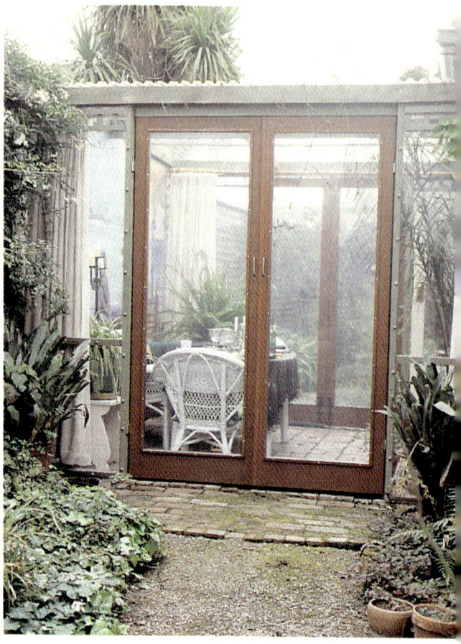

Provide the gardener with a user-friendly microclimate—a conservatory for a frost-tender gardener.

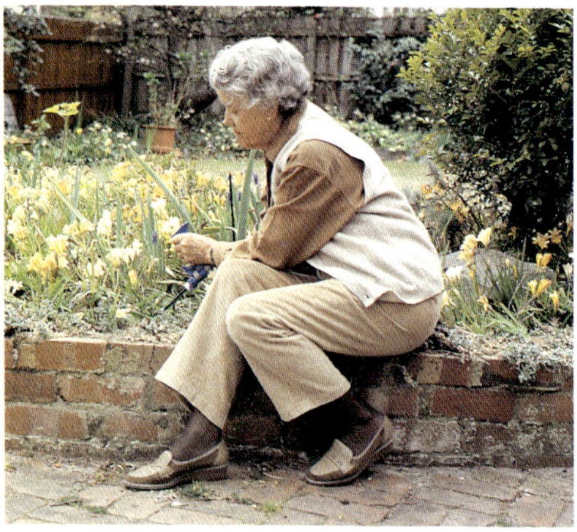

62

Above centre: *A young rose bush after a year in a root control bag. This plant was dug up and moved during an extended hot spell; it has happily established in its new home, and* right *a close-up of the root control bag with above plant.*

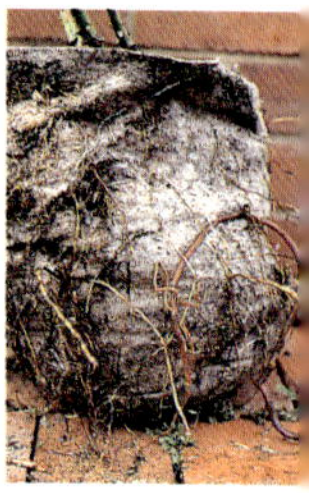

Left: *A low raised bed can be used as a seat while working in the garden. Care should be taken to ensure the height is correct.*

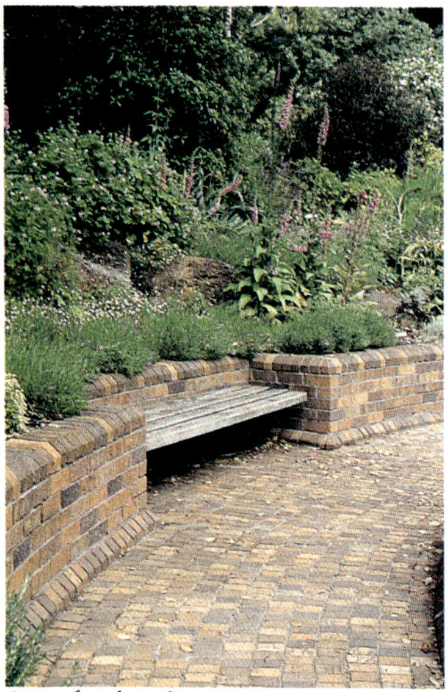

63

A garden bench set into a retaining wall in the Herb Garden. The paved surfaces give year-round easy access.

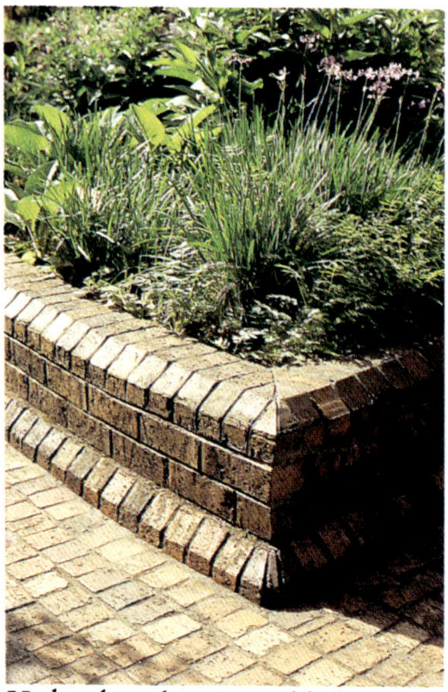

64

Herbs planted in a raised bed in the Herb Garden at the Royal Melbourne Botanic Gardens.

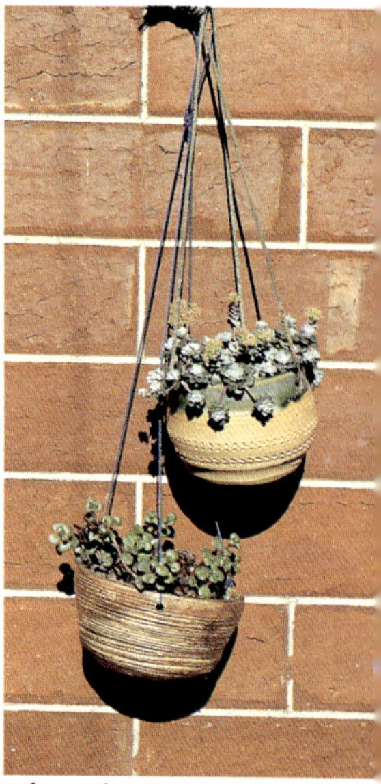

These dainty succulents are jewel-like in their tiny hanging pots.

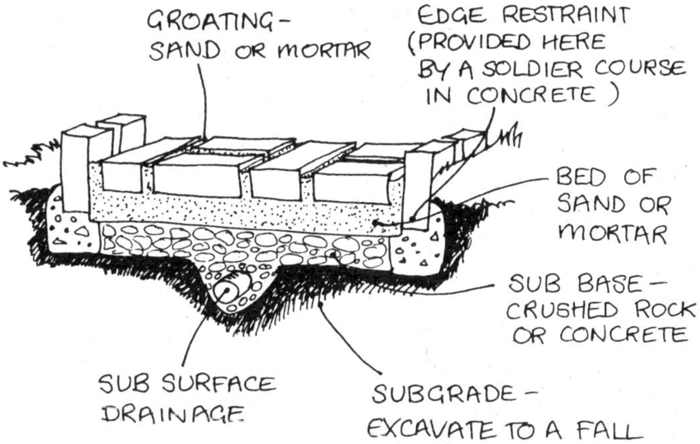

Paving profile.

Note that the roots of some trees are highly invasive or have large buttress roots, and can disrupt hard surfaces. If you are paving near such trees, use a suitable root barrier to restrict root growth in the direction of the paving.

Concrete

Concrete was a fairly uninteresting and 'unsympathetic' surface in the garden until the arrival of a number of modern treatments; however, its sheer practicality and hard wearingness have found it a place in many homes. Smooth concrete is too slippery for safety; a broomed finish is a much safer option. Here the surface is brushed with a hard broom before the concrete has set to give it a textured top layer that offers far greater traction. So too does concrete that has had the surface aggregate exposed. This is done by washing the surface free of the cement mixture before it has fully hardened, thereby exposing the aggregate.

Concrete in its native state is a bright, glary material no matter what the surface texture. A vast array of colours are available for tinting the concrete. These may be used to colour the entire slab or else they can be simply applied as a surface render. The latter alternative is, of course, far less enduring that the former. A coloured render can be applied to an existing concrete slab, although a thicker layer will be needed than when treating a new slab. Judicious colour selection, combined with brooming or exposed aggregate, give a surface that is both safe and which will be less harsh in the garden environment.

'Faux Brick' is a new processing technique that can be used to give concrete an appearance very like many traditional paving materials such as brick, tiles and stone; ersatz slate, cobblestones, fishscale fans, herringbone and circular brick pavings are possible, to name but a few. It is surprisingly convincing, both as regards the colours and the patterns, and may be acceptable to many people who would not otherwise consider using concrete in the garden. The final step in the 'fauxing' with many of the patterns involves the application of a 'scratch coat' which gives the concrete a roughened texture, thereby increasing its slip resistance. In the case of the stone- and tile-like patterns, a smooth trowelled finish would usually be done for the sake of authenticity. The scratch coat can easily be applied to these patterns to make them low-slip, but this will need to be specified at the outset to the tradesperson carrying out the work. This treatment has been around in Australia for only a relatively short time and has not been thoroughly assessed for its suitability for all situations; however, it does *appear* to offer good slip resistance. It is certainly marketed as such (though that, unfortunately, is not always something one can go by). The surface is long-lasting and virtually maintenance-free unless it has been laid where moss and algae are able to grow. Then, of course, it should be scrubbed with the algaecide, usually a copper-based mixture that will kill algae, moss and slime.

'Faux Brick' paving is something that needs to be done by a professional; it involves two separate surfacing procedures and the use of stencils. Both the application of subtly varied colours *and* the laying of the often complex stencils require some considerable degree of technical expertise, and at this stage the ingredients are not available to the do-it-yourself-er. The finish is quite thick, too thick to go over existing concrete slabs, and needs to be applied as a slab is being poured. It is also something that is only available through a limited number of licensed contractors. There are 'cowboys' out there offering the product but in fact they are actually only able to supply stamped concrete in various patterns. The finish of the stamped concrete is nowhere near as slip-resistant as that of the 'Faux Brick'; neither is the appearance of the stamped concrete convincingly like those of the materials it seeks to imitate, thus it is important to locate the real thing. The surest way to do this is through your State branch of the National Ready Mix Concrete Association (NRMCA).

Existing concrete slabs can be made safer by surface treatments, including one that can give an appearance similar to traditional unit paving materials, which again will require a skilled tradesperson for its application.

Laying a concrete slab There are many useful books available with instructions on laying a concrete slab; the following is intended as a brief guide to the work involved so that you can decide whether or not you should even contemplate DIY-ing. Laying a slab requires timber form-work. As with brick paving, the topsoil must be removed; any drainage problems must be attended to at this stage and if the subgrade is unstable then a footing of crushed rock will need to be laid. The thickness of the slab will vary according to the stability of the soil and the traffic the area is to carry; correctly installed reinforcing and expansion joints may well be necessary to control cracking. Ready-mixed cement brought in from suppliers is normally used for all but the smallest of jobs.

Tiles

Non-slip tiles made from materials such as clay or slate are available.

What has been a voluntary code of practice regarding slip resistance standards is in the process of becoming law. As with paving bricks, a minimum Coefficient of Friction of 0.4 is required for slip-resistant outdoor tiles. Those that are suitable for around swimming pools will usually be the most slip-resistant. If you have trouble obtaining the information you require for a particular tile, contact the manufacturers directly.

Cut stone

Natural stone is a beautiful though expensive material in the garden. As with tiles, the voluntary code of practice on slip resistance standards is gradually becoming law, and some larger suppliers already evaluate their stones for slip resistance; however, some smaller suppliers may not do so routinely; in such a case it is advisable to change your choice to a supplier who does.

Large paved areas — Patios and terraces

An area may be paved to allow its use as an outdoor eating area, as a utility area for the clothesline or the rubbish bins, or as a quiet spot for a garden seat. Good siting is crucial if these areas are to fulfill their intended purpose: an outdoor entertainment area should be located near to or adjoining the kitchen, a utilities area should be easily reached from the house, yet tucked away from view. This part of the design process will be dealt with later in this chapter.

Always attend to drainage — remember to slope the area and to install a drainage pit which connects up to the stormwater system. Avoid sloping the paving towards the house — a paved area will collect a surprising amount of water and in case the storm water drainage fails (heaven forbid, but it has been known to happen), the water should be able to drain somewhere other than into the kitchen. If your paving abutts the house, make sure that it does not block air vents or bury the damp course. If for any reason you are unable to excavate down to the recommended level, for example, if you are laying brick paving over an existing slab, then do not bring the paving right up to the house if it will interfere with ventilation or cover up the damp course — always allow sufficient space for air circulation: a gap of 20 cm (8″) is recommended.

Paths

Paths are constructed using the same methods as larger areas, but some additional factors must be considered. Paths should reflect the traffic patterns within an area wherever possible, that is the paths should be laid where we would naturally want to walk. This is usually the shortest path between A and B and, unless there is some problem with doing so, this is usually the best course to take. Paths should be wide enough for people and equipment to pass along comfortably — 1 metre (3′3″) wide for one person and 1.2 metres (3′11″) for two people or someone who is in a wheelchair or who uses a walking frame.

Edges should be clearly visible or indicated by a tactile marker such as a raised edge if this is appropriate. Paths should be level across their width, apart from the 1:60 slope that must be allowed for water to run off. Steeply sloping paths should be avoided—a slope of 1:20 is considered negotiable by most people. If the land is steep then consider building the path across the natural slope. If this is either impractical or would be visually jarring, then steps or a ramp with landings at regular intervals should be installed. Handrails should also be used on all difficult sections of a path.

Steps

Steps are usually made out of the same materials as the other paved areas. Proper construction with these materials requires a concrete base and therefore formwork is necessary. The gradient of these steps will be determined by the dimensions of the risers (the vertical part of a step) and the tread (the horizontal part you put your foot on); these, in turn, should be determined by the gait of the person who must use them. A riser of 180 mm (7″) is the *maximum* for those with a normal gait, while for those who need to take it easy, a maximum of 150 mm (6″) is advised. If in doubt, seek advice from a health professional or your State ILC. The tread should be at least 300 mm (1′) deep. A wide tread and a shallow riser give a gentle climb. A comfortable relationship between the riser and the tread is given by the formula:

2x (Riser in mm) + Tread in mm = 650–675 mm
[2x (Riser in ins) + Tread in ins = 25.5–26.5 inches]

Steps with open risers, that is, vertical gaps between the horizontal treads, are a risky proposition, as is a spiral staircase. A single step all on its own should never be used, it is all too easily overlooked. If your stairway is long, a landing should be provided every 5 or 6 steps. It is often recommended that the tread be made to overhang the riser slightly to create a cunning little shadow that will further define each step. This protrusion can be dangerous, especially to those whose eyesight is poor or who have mobility problems—finish the tread *flush* with the riser. If the steps are to be used by someone with severe visual impairment, a strip of a contrasting light colour such as white or yellow, or else a strip with a tell-tale change of texture—a ‘tactile indicator’—are recommended. These strips should be at least 25 mm (1″) wide; additional tactile indicators on the top and the bottom step are recommended.

Ramps

Ramps are easier to negotiate than steps in many cases. Whether they are preferred to steps will depend on the user—for those in a wheelchair a ramp will obviously be the first choice; those with a walking frame or walking stick may also prefer a ramp, though some find gentle steps easier to negotiate. Ramps should be of a generous width—1.5 metres is desirable. The maximum gradient of 1:14 is recommended. Ramps should be supplied with a handrail and should be made of a non-slip material—the steeper the ramp, the higher the slip resistance rating needs to be; a build-up of momentum when coming down a ramp is both dangerous and alarming.

Handrails

Handrails should be installed in all areas where there is a major change in levels, that is, on all ramps, steps or steep sections of a path. They should, of course, be strong and well constructed; the rails should be smooth and comfortable to hold—a diameter of 50 mm (2″) gives a comfortable grip for most. They should also be constructed of materials that do not change temperature to any great extent—metal handrails will become too hot to hold in the summer sun, and wet and chilly in the winter. Those who are concerned that the handrails will add too institutional an air to their garden should consider using wood for the rail—take a look around public parks and gardens where handrails have been installed to see what materials you find acceptable. Wooden handrails may require some maintenance to keep them free of splinters. A handrail should extend beyond the end of the steps or ramp by at least the width of one tread rather than end abruptly. This way users will not have to cope with the change in slope unassisted. A downward curve towards the end of the rail provides a tactile clue to the visually impaired and can give the handrail a pleasing 'finished' appearance.

Outdoor lighting

Lighting can extend the usefulness of an outdoor area as well as improving night-time safety for paths, steps and other transit areas. Increased sensitivity to glare means that older gardeners must be careful with placement of lighting. For preference, lights should shine *down* on the area to be illuminated, and be positioned so that shadows are not cast in a way that may mislead us. Any low level lighting should either be hooded or fitted with diffusers to prevent light shining directly into the eyes.

Exterior lighting is an art-form, and any gardener who truly wants to get the most out of their garden at night would do well to utilise the skills of a specialist in the field. If you decide to DIY, make sure you buy your lighting from a reputable manufacturer, and be sure to follow their safety instructions to the letter. Experimenting with torches before installation can help find the best positions for the lights in the area to be illuminated.

Raised Garden Beds

For many of us, it is in actually *working* in the garden, getting our hands dirty tending our plants, that much of the joy is to be found; it would be a sore loss if we could no longer do this. Sadly, this has been the lot of some gardeners who are unable to work in conventional gardens, whether because of back problems, arthritis or a stroke. Raised garden beds allow easy access to the soil surface for those who have difficulty reaching the ground, whatever the cause of the difficulties. Used extensively in horticultural therapy gardens for this reason, raised beds also offer the advantage of bringing the plants closer to eye level, allowing their pleasures to be more easily savoured. Thus they are a boon both to those who cannot bend and those who are partially sighted.

Raised garden beds may be free-standing structures which allow access from all sides. They may also be built behind a retaining wall, or with one wall abutting an existing structure such as a boundary fence. In these last cases they cannot be reached all the way around. The dimensions of the bed will be determined by the needs of the user; both the height of the gardener and their disability will have a bearing on this.

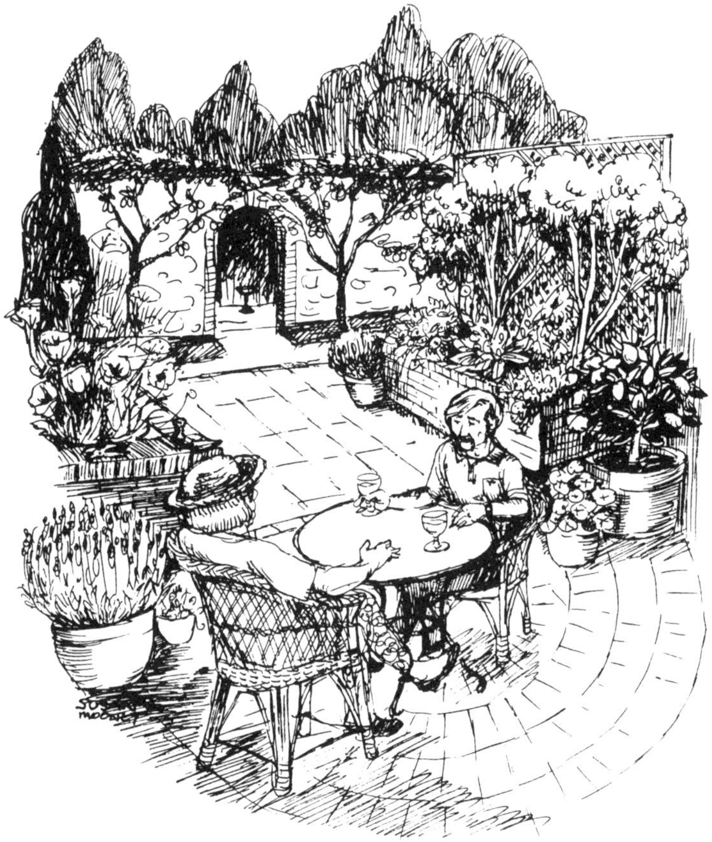

The recommended height for standing users is 710 mm (2′4″) for those with leg or back injury, and 865 mm (2′10″) for those with difficulties in bending; 610 mm (2′) is the recommended height for wheelchair users. However, recommendations are only approximate; the *exact* height needed should always be determined, either by 'trial and error' with a mock-up of the bed, or with the help of a health professional such as an occupational therapist. When the bed can only be reached from one side, then its width should only be that distance that can be comfortably reached—usually about 600 mm (2′). Where there is access from both sides, the bed can be twice this width. If desired, extra features such as a toe recess, hand rails, tool rests and seating can be incorporated.

Wheelchair users will usually need to work side-on to the beds. T-shaped beds (trays on legs—the tray is the top of the T, the legs, the downward stroke) have sometimes been used, but to accommodate the arms of a wheelchair underneath the tray, the tray will usually be too high to allow the user to garden comfortably, and too shallow to grow most plants.

The beds can be made in most of the usual materials used for garden structures, such as brick, timber and concrete. The shape and the length of the beds are a matter of personal preference for the gardener; they can be built to virtually any shape and can be made to fit into any layout and garden style. Rectangular beds are the simplest to construct and the most common; L-shaped and cruciform beds are only slightly more difficult to build and can make an aesthetic contribution to the overall garden design without sacrificing accessibility. Curved beds are yet another alternative but require a good deal more technical know-how. A raised bed can be used to enclose a paved courtyard most effectively, and for those gardening in a small space, they can be employed to make the area seem larger than it is.

Raised beds must be rigid and stable. However, providing access to the soil surface is the 'raison d'être' of the raised bed; this limits the materials that can be used to those which are sufficiently narrow in cross-section. Thus a rock wall, especially one with a set-back (a backward lean), would be unsuitable. Safety is also a consideration. Some users may need to lean or slump against the sides so walls and the foundations of the raised beds should be built according to the engineering principles used in the construction of retaining walls.

Drainage is usually unnecessary in the raised beds where they drain directly onto the soil, particularly when 'leaky' materials such as timber are used for the beds. However, the inclusion of drainage at the base of the design will be necessary when the beds are built over a hard surface; as it is neither difficult nor expensive to include drainage in the beds this should perhaps be done with solid materials, for example, concrete and brick, that lend themselves to a build up of hydrostatic pressure. To provide weep-holes in brick beds, mortar is simply omitted between occasional bricks near the base. With a concrete bed, provision for weep-holes will need to be made in the form prior to pouring. A watering system should be installed in the beds at the time of construction.

Free-standing raised beds

Timber raised beds

Timber is often used in the garden because of its colour, texture, and the feeling that it looks well with living plant material. For a raised garden bed either a rot resistant hardwood such as red gum or jarrah or else treated pine should be used; these have a life of around twenty-five years. Sawn planks, railway sleepers or treated pine logs are all suitable for the walling; the sleepers and logs are rather more expensive than the planks.

Construction details Because of the variability of the lateral pressures exerted by different soil types, it is difficult to make precise recommendations for timber beds; however, to ensure a timber bed is safe and structurally sound, observe the following:

—In a stable soil, support posts should be set in concrete footings to 600 mm (24″) or else in a 50/50 dry mix of cement and earth to the same depth as the height of the wall; for unstable soils they should be either set in the cement-earth mix a further 40 per cent, or else set in concrete footings. If unsure of your soil type or the type of footing you should be using, the engineers department of your local shire or council will be able to help you. A permit may be required from your council for a raised bed, usually for those over 1 metre (3′ 3″)—enquire *before* you start.

—Use square timbers for the support posts; these offer the greatest resistance to bending and present a large face to the soil.

—Always use good quality, rot-resistant wood for the whole construction.

—Bolt the wood in place—do not use screws—using galvanised bolts.

—For long, parallel walls, internal bracing posts or tie-backs should be used every 1–1.5 metres (3′ 3″–5′).

Additional drainage is unnecessary with timber because water can escape through gaps and pores in the material; indeed with treated pine logs it may be necessary to line the beds with a semi-permeable material to prevent loss of soil through cracks.

A toe recess makes a raised bed more ergonomically sound. If you're not sure what is meant by this, or of its value, take a look at a well-designed modern kitchen bench or appliance. They will have a recess at their base to allow the user to get right up close when working. A toe recess is easily incorporated in a wooden bed, though with other materials it can make the design more complicated.

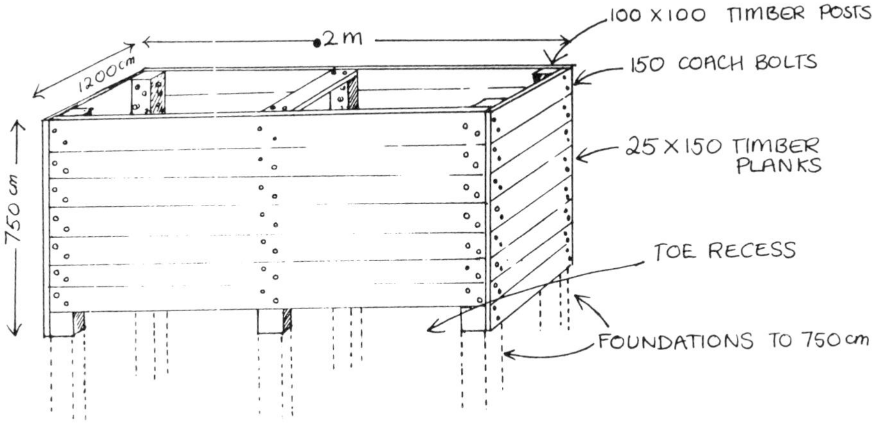

Timber raised garden bed.

Brick wall thickness for raised bed.

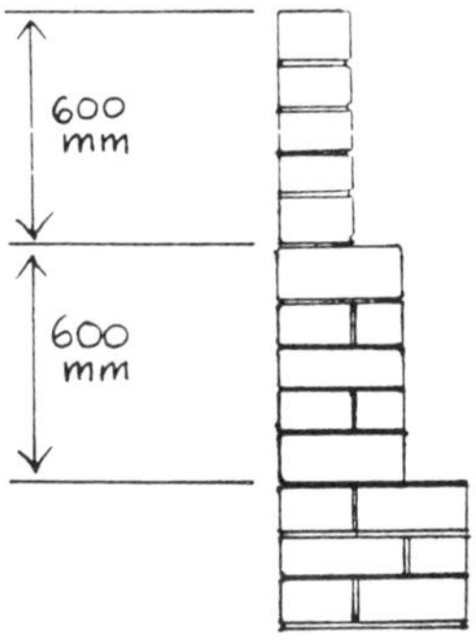

Brick raised beds

Brick has a more formal appearance than timber but blends well with most plant materials. It is the obvious choice where the house is made of bricks or where bricks are used elsewhere in the garden.

Concrete foundations are required for all brick raised beds. The depth of the footings should be the same as the thickness of the wall or 250 mm (10″), whichever is the greater; the width of the footings should be twice the thickness of the wall or the thickness of the wall plus 300 mm (1′), whichever is the greater. The footing should be reinforced with trench mesh. If this is not done properly, the footing will break up in time. An appropriate text or expert should be consulted.

The thickness and the weight of a wall contributes to the strength of the wall. A double thickness of bricks will increase strength, as will the construction of brick piers to act as buttresses. As the pressure exerted by the soil decreases towards the top of the beds, the wall thickness can be stepped. To do this, the wall should be divided into 600 mm (2′) units *starting from the top*. If the wall is to be built without buttresses, then each successive unit, beneath the top unit of one brick's thickness, should be at least half a brick thicker than the one above.

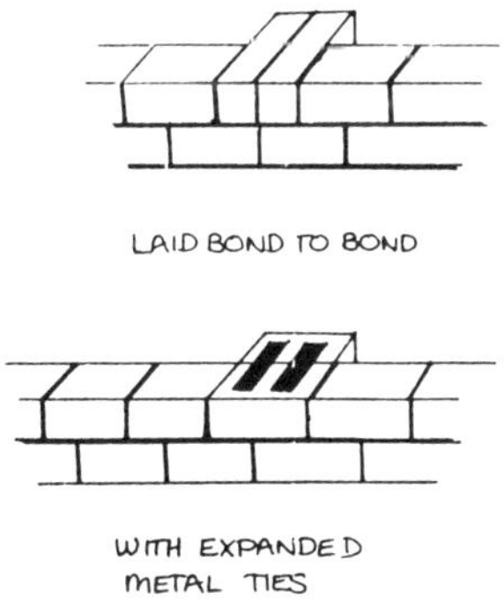

Brick piers.

If buttresses are to be used to achieve the necessary strength, these should occur at intervals at least as often as twice the height of the wall and never less than once every 2 metres (6′7″). The pier should be bonded to the wall when constructed so that its bricks lie through the wall and at right angles to the wall bonding; if the bricks in the pier are to lie parallel to those of the wall, then they should be tied to the wall using expanded metal ties. The piers should be constructed on the *inside* of the bed, rather than protruding outwards, for reasons of safety and access. In a raised bed whose walls are less than 2 metres, the end walls will act as buttresses.

Drainholes should be incorporated in the bottom course of bricks at intervals of no more than 1 metre. This can be done by omitting the mortar between two adjacent bricks or by building in lengths of plastic or earthenware pipes on the inside of the bed. The pipes should protrude through but not beyond the walling, or there will be a lot of unnecessary suffering of unsuspecting shins.

The top course of bricks of a brick raised bed can be capped with bricks laid side-on to provide a resting surface for tools and plants if so desired.

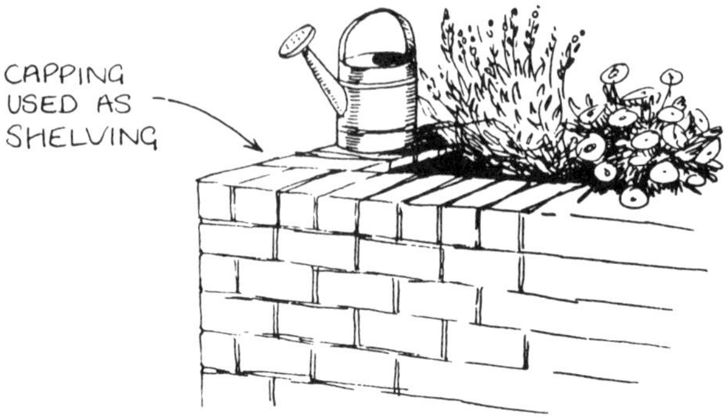

Capping used as a shelf.

Concrete raised beds

Concrete is very often rejected as a building material for raised planters because of its 'unsympathetic' appearance. It is more expensive than brick but can be very long lasting; its appearance can be greatly improved by treatments such as painting, applying a coloured render or facing the surface with tiles or a thin veneer of stone. Furthermore, because concrete is poured where it is to stand, complicated shapes are possible and idiosyncratic requirements are more easily met. A wooden form must be built for the bed, with foundations as for brick. Forms for toe holes and any other small requirement can be made using strong cardboard boxes bent to the appropriate dimensions. Drainage holes will also be needed, and should be provided for during pouring by inserting pipes near the base and spaced as for brick beds. Again, finish the pipes flush with the wall to avoid skinning shins. Trench mesh should be used in the foundations, and reinforcement may be necessary in the walls; an engineer should be consulted while still in the planning phase.

Raised beds from other materials

Other materials such as concrete blocks or stone are also suitable building materials for raised beds and may be the choice of some gardeners. Be aware that thick walls will limit access to the bed, so choose your material accordingly.

Raised beds from retaining walls

Many older gardeners would perhaps choose not to live on a steeply sloping site. However, a house set in the hills may be some peoples' dream, despite the inconvenience, or they may already live on such a block and do not wish to move on retirement. Retaining walls help to create flat, functional terraces on a steep block and can also be used to make raised garden beds.

The pressure exerted on a retaining wall by the soil on a steep incline can be considerable, as can the hydrostatic pressure if water is allowed to build up behind it. Thus it is vital that the wall be structurally sound. Any retaining wall that is over 600 mm (2′) *or* that is built in an area where the soil is prone to any movement—'reactive'—will need to be designed by an engineer. Again, check with your local council on this.

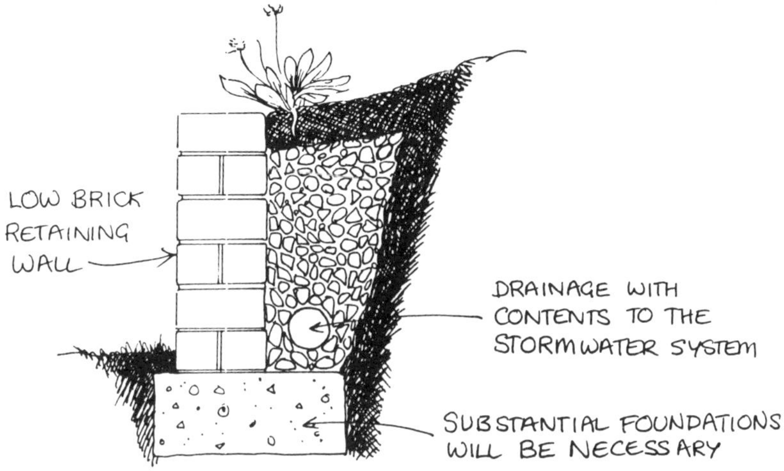

Profile of a retaining wall.

Siting a raised bed—drainage, paving

There is little point in investing the time and money in building a raised bed if the ground around is often too wet and soggy, too rough or too slippery to allow comfortable use. Give careful thought to siting the bed—is your chosen spot really the best, or are there other sites that

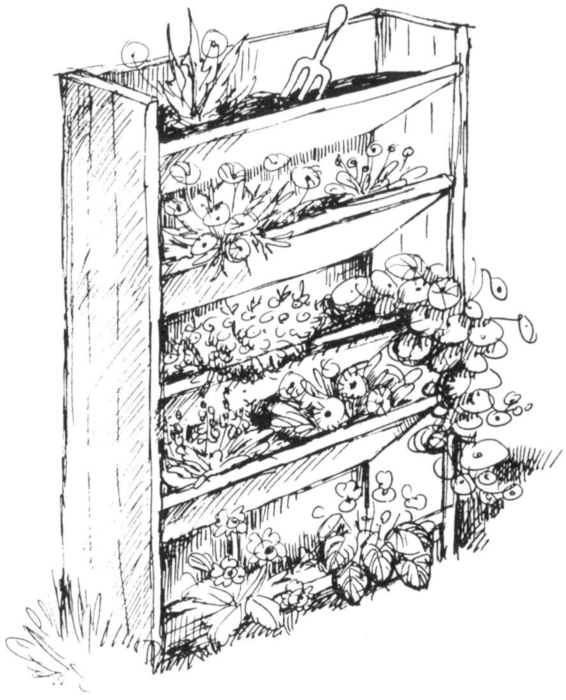

Planting shelves.

would be sunnier/drier/more easily reached? If the bed must be built in a spot where some form of drainage is required, then this must be attended to *first* before anything else goes down on the site. Paving the area will increase its usability many times over and should be done for any gardener with mobility problems.

Planting in raised containers

A cheap and cheerful alternative to raised garden beds is offered by planting in containers on a raised surface. This could be done with pots up on a table, growing things in window boxes or hanging baskets, or by gardening in purpose-built shelving. These last alternatives are particularly useful to those who must garden in small spaces. Planting shelves further extend the gardening possible for those who are restricted to just a balcony or courtyard, for they allow a range of annual food crops or flowers to be grown in a very small space. Gardening in containers is dealt with in detail in Chapter 6.

Climate Modification

We often put great effort into giving our plants the microclimate they need to do their best. Shade-lovers are planted under spreading boughs, prairie plants given an open border, tender woodland plants awarded a sheltered site in dappled light. Just as often we neglect the fact that we humans, too, need favourable microclimates in order to flourish. We need a sunny spot to sit and feel the spring awaken our winter-dulled senses, we need deep shade to escape the summer heat, a gentle breeze to refresh in the humidity of the tropics. We need suitable microclimates to work and to play in our gardens, and these we can build into our outdoors environment.

Windbreaks

A well-designed windbreak can shelter the area behind it for up to ten times its height. This can be important not only for protection from cold winter winds but also from the harsh, hot summer winds that blow in from our desert interior.

Solid fences are not the best windbreaks; solid barriers cause turbulence and can give us a worse problem than we started with. Research in agriculture and forestry has shown that the best shelterbelts are wide plantings of trees of a variety of different heights and forms. A shelterbelt should oppose the prevailing wind and so should be positioned accordingly, curving around toward the ends to deal with variations in the wind direction that is usual. Of course, those of us living in the cities or suburbs will seldom be able to plant the wide belts that will give us maximum protection, nor will we be able to avoid unbroken paling fences. However, we can still do something to break the worst of the offending winds by observing the following points:

Greatest protection is given to the area immediately on the leeward side of a shelterbelt and is a function of its height.

Planting trees with a variety of different shapes and forms will break up the wind but avoid turbulence. Densely foliated trees with foliage on low branches offer the best protection, but even the bare boughs of a deciduous tree in winter will still filter the wind, reducing its force considerably. This may be important where shelter from seasonal winds might be seemingly incompatible with light requirements in a dwelling—either yours or your neighbour's. A windbreak will start to deflect the wind before the wind actually hits it and so will offer some protection on the windward side. Step down your windbreak by planting tall shrubs and trees on the leeward side where possible; take the variation in wind directions into account and plant your windbreak 'around corners' where you are able.

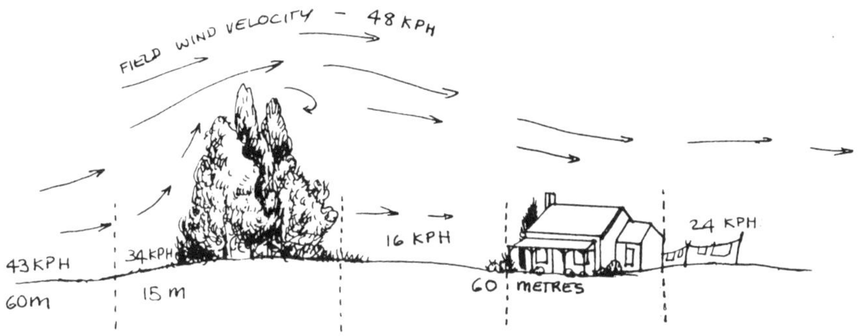

Area sheltered by windbreak showing the degree of reduction—plant trees of different heights and shapes.

For a very small garden, a solid wall will provide adequate wind protection; the turbulence this barrier causes will happen somewhere else beyond the garden. Where a fence is the only windbreak available for a larger garden, a broken structure such as a picket or woven fence will filter the wind without adding to the turbulence. If this is incompatible

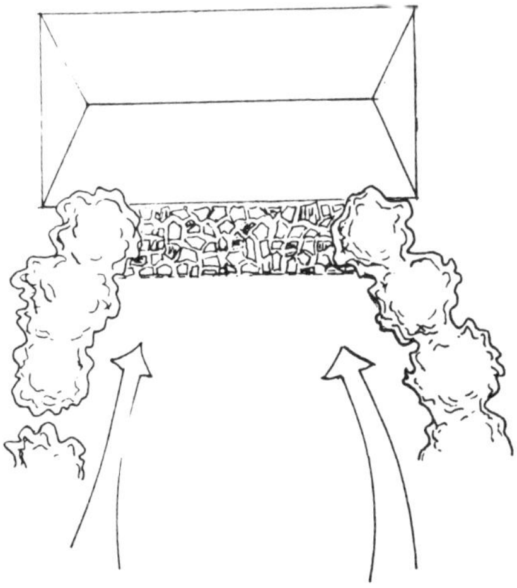

Directing a flow of air to a specific area.

with privacy or noise reduction requirements, then perhaps a mixed planting of slender trees along the fenceline could be accommodated. Country gardeners should consult the Department of Agriculture for suitable windbreak trees, while city gardeners can choose from the trees and shrubs noted as wind resistant from the lists in Chapter 6.

Where a breeze is needed for personal comfort in the house or an outside area, trees and shrubs can be used to funnel moving air to the desired spot. Air turbulence is complex and a through-draft can be created by bouncing air currents off obstacles some distance away or by creating a 'clearing in the forest' situation; those with the space to try such schemes should contact their local Energy Information Centre for information. For most gardeners, hedging or a line of isolated shrubs or trees will best serve this purpose.

Noise reduction

Where noise is a problem, a solid barrier will be required, the higher the better. Generally, a fence of more than 2 metres (6′ 7″) in height will require a special permit from the council. For a fence to provide an effective noise barrier it must be of solid construction with no gaps or open letter boxes. High density materials such as bricks and concrete blocks are the most effective for reducing noise transmission, however, 20 mm pine planking and fibre-cement sheets are dense enough to bring about significant noise reduction.

A noise barrier must be placed to break the line of sight between the source of the noise and the area to be shielded. Where traffic is the problem, far better noise reduction is achieved if your near neighbours can be persuaded to erect tall fences as well. Where neighbours *are* the problem, a taller barrier may be necessary. Some councils will permit such a wall *inside* your fenceline, but it may mean sacrificing a 60 cm (2′) strip of your land along the shared boundary.

Light and shade

Plants moderate the sunlight that reaches earth. Nature has designed them to absorb, reflect and filter the sun with superb efficiency; how fitting it is that they should form our first line of defence against harsh extremes in the garden. Built structures can perform these functions too, but perhaps do so best when combined with plants.

Light and shade are basic elements in the garden and great care should be spent in getting them right. Not only can they make an enormous difference to our comfort, they can also affect our safety outdoors. Skin cancer remains a major problem in Australia—at present we have the highest incidence of skin cancer in the world and two out of every three Australians will develop a skin cancer at some stage in their lives. More people get sunburnt in their garden each weekend than anywhere else outdoors—more than on the beach, more than on the cricket pitch or on the tennis court. It is vital that we use sunscreen, wear hats and cover-up clothing when we go out in the sun. It is vital, too, that we sunscape our gardens so that shaded areas for activity and rest are available when they are needed.

As we age, we become slower at adjusting to changes in the level of illumination, thus if we pass abruptly from a dimly lit area into a bright one, we may find ourselves temporarily blinded. On its own, this may be merely disconcerting and uncomfortable, but if combined with a mobility problem, difficulties with balance or visual impairment it may have serious consequences.

Transition areas where we pass from an indoor to an outdoor environment should be a half-way house with regard to illumination to allow our eyes to adjust to the different levels of light. Entryways can be lightly shaded with lattice; climbers can be grown to give a denser shade.

Pergolas can be built onto houses to shade the entrances or to form shaded walkways over paths. Pergolas can provide shade with the addition of climbing plants, tightly woven fabric, or carefully angled slats to block out the summer sun but admit the lower rays of autumn and spring.

Well-positioned trees can perform the same function. Trees evoke a powerful response in most of us and their presence in a garden can add much to its strength; they are rightly the first thing that most gardeners will consider when planting out their garden. Trees are valuable not only for their beauty but for cool, still, shade that lies beneath their canopy. A mature shade tree creates an almost magical environment beneath its boughs, where it is cool and moist and peaceful through even the most merciless of summers. However, they are an altogether more complicated proposition than a built structure for shading a particular part of a house. For a start, a tree must grow to a considerable size before it starts providing shade where it is needed. In most cases this means it is years, even decades before this end is achieved. Trees must be carefully selected, too, for their compatibility with house foundations and paving. Some commonly planted trees such as liquidambar and weeping willow are disastrous when planted near buildings and should be avoided anywhere near the house.

Not all trees have leaf canopies that will provide significant shade at ground level. The size of the leaves, the angle at which they are held and the branching pattern of the trees together will determine the amount of shade that a tree provides. Many Australian natives have evolved strategies for avoiding the full strength of the sun, such as holding their leaves vertically, and so cast little shadow. Broad-leafed exotics are often the best choice for providing shade. A list of suitable shade trees for both near the house and in the open is given in the next chapter.

Pergolas, arbours and gazebos

A pergola at maturity forms a tunnel of dappled light and greenery, with optional delights of flowers, fruit, or seasonal colour. Whether free-standing or adjoining the house, it has the potential to be one of the most ornamental and usable structures in the garden. If paved, it can serve as an outdoor living area or a functional walkway, or it can act visually as a divider within the garden. With the addition of a seat, it becomes a resting place, with a table, it becomes a dining-room, a chess hall, a studio, a propagation area. Planted with deciduous climbers, a pergola will offer shade in the summer; in late autumn and early spring the cover will be sparse, allowing the light to penetrate below.

Pergolas consist of vertical posts or pillars which support horizontal beams. Rafters are attached to the beams, lying across them at right angles. Battens can, if desired, be attached to the rafters to provide further shade. Cloth can be used to provide some shade until the plants have grown enough to protect us. Use either a shadecloth with a rating of *no less than 90 per cent* (lower ratings are for plants, not for people), or else use a tightly woven fabric which casts a dense shade. Be aware though that a cloth acts like sun screen lotion—it increases the time that we can stay outside, but eventually we will burn. While the question is still being researched, it is possible that because plants actually absorb UV rays, they create better quality shade than fabrics. Still, by combining these treatments, a shade-versatile space can be created.

Pergolas are commonly made of timber, though the pillars may be brick or stone with timber beams and rafters, or the entire construction may be metal. A pergola can be attached to a house, in which case the posts adjacent to the house may be omitted. Most councils require a permit for a pergola, so be prepared to submit your plans before you start building.

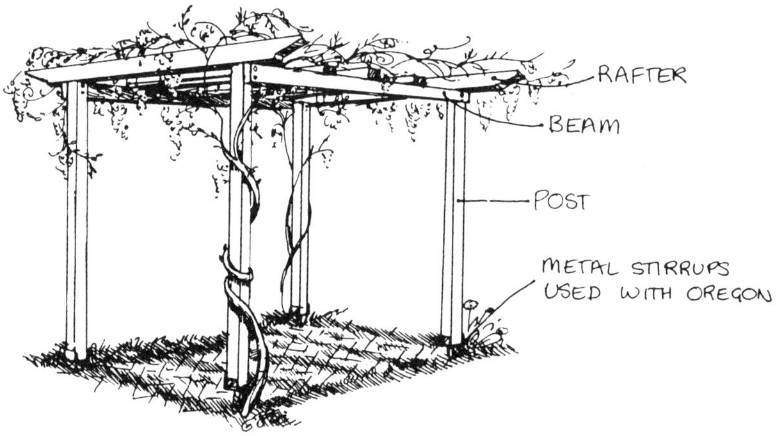

Pergola structure.

A pergola must support a considerable weight as the climbers grow and so it must be strongly built and well constructed. Rot-resistant materials should, of course, be used. Oregon is often used for timber pergolas as it is relatively inexpensive; however, as oregon will rot in the ground, galvanised metal stirrups should be used to set it into its foundations. These stirrups are made specifically for this task and are available from builders' suppliers and larger hardware stores; they can easily be disguised by a planting if they are found unsightly. The overhead cover will offer little protection from the rain, so unless a pergola is purely to provide visual accent it should be paved underneath or have some form of suitable hard surface. A pergola may not be maintenance-free: climbers will need training, tying in and pruning, moss and algae may enjoy the conditions created underneath and will need to be removed, fallen leaves will be slippery underfoot and must be attended to. In return, a pergola offers months of congenial outdoor living space that can be custom-made to a gardener's needs.

An arbour is essentially a smaller, more intimate version of the pergola. The use of arbours in European gardens dates back at least to mediaeval times; then they may have been constructed entirely by intertwining the long, flexible canes of a climber, or they may have been carpenter-built. The living arbours were often formed from climbing roses, but these are seldom the most user-friendly of plants for an arbour or pergola. Again, look to the next chapter for plants to suit this purpose.

A gazebo or summer house gives all-weather protection from sun and rain. Because they are roofed with building materials rather than living plants they will remain shaded throughout the year. They may be open structures, merely columns supporting a roof, or they may be enclosed on all but one side. They may be as simple or as fanciful as you will and can be a highly ornamental garden feature. They can be graced by a planting or stand alone on their architectural merits.

Water as a cooling agent

Water is inherently therapeutic and may be included in a garden purely for its aesthetic appeal. Whether still and reflective in bowl or pond, or rushing and gleaming in fountain or stream, water can soothe and delight. Water can also act as an evaporative 'air conditioner' in the garden, cooling its immediate surrounds and the areas that lie downwind. It has been used for this purpose with great skill in Mediterranean gardens and those of the Middle East for centuries.

The greater the amount of water exposed to the air, the greater will be its cooling effect. Thus a fountain which keeps a constant supply of cool water running and spraying into a small pool may cool to the same degree as a larger area of still water. In either case, water is to be found cooling gardens in areas that experience hot, dry conditions in summer. In the arid regions of Persia and southern Spain, water is used to cool and to irrigate the garden as well as for its symbolic value. It is used in fountains and runnels, in canals and in pools.

Water may be used in both formal and informal gardens. It is equally at home in the magnificence of Versailles or the Taj Mahal, or the modest serenity of a Japanese garden or a small bush block. Still water provides a perfect breeding ground for mosquitoes in a warm climate. To avoid this happening, a garden pool or pond should be stocked with fish to eat the mosquito larvae and water plants to oxygenate the water for the fish—either this, or the water should be kept circulating to keep it fresh and mosquito-free. In most parts of Australia we must conserve water and so we will need to recycle that which we use in our water features; small, almost noiseless pumps are available for this purpose.

Water will attract birds, as well as desirable insects such as damsel- and dragon-flies. A raised pool will allow us near the water surface, to experience both the cooling effect and the delights of the water up close. A wide capping on the side of the pool will allow us to sit right at the edge, or seating can be placed at its side.

Permanent Seating

All gardens need permanent seating. On a garden seat we can sit and contemplate our small piece of paradise, take in all the sights, the sounds, the fragrances of the garden, drink in the beauty of it all. A garden seat calls to us to come and sit, to take our ease in the cool of the shade or bask in the warmth of spring. A well-placed seat can transform the garden from a place to work or pass through into a place worthy of our full attention, a place to be experienced.

A garden seat should be used, too, to rest on while we are working. There should be good, solid, seating placed near all the areas where we spend time working—a vegetable patch, a propagation area, or a spot with container-grown plants are all likely candidates for a garden bench. It is important that a seat be stable, comfortable, and be there when you need it. Fold-up seats miss out hands down on all of these points—too light for stability, they frequently move as we place ourselves down in

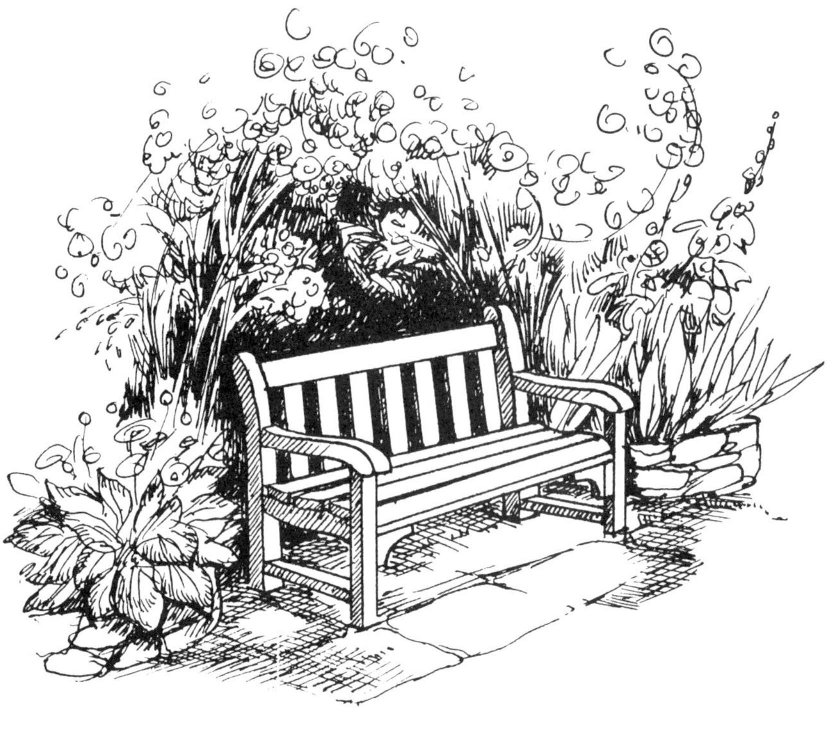

A comfortable seat in a garden setting.

them, fold up when we least expect it, and furthermore are usually locked in the garden shed when we need them most! For safety, a garden seat should be solid and well constructed; it should be placed on ground that is firm and even. For comfort, it should have a backrest for support, arms to help with getting up and down, and be of a suitable height. A ground-to-seat measurement of 480 mm (19″) is a generally user-friendly height, and a good deep seat of 480 mm often suits. Before you buy, sit in a seat for as long as you can and get in and out of it several times. If it seems to suit you, then consider.

A handsome seat makes a splendid garden feature. Many beautiful garden seats are available, ranging in spirit from the simple charm of a rustic wooden bench to the exquisite delicacy of a Victorian wrought iron 'chaise'. The prices range, too, from below one hundred dollars for a mass-produced seat to as high as you like for a hand-crafted job. 'Cheap and cheerful' garden seats are readily available from hardware stores and furniture suppliers. If they are strongly made and comfortable, they may be equally useful whether assigned to a focal point in the garden or an out-of-the-way high maintenance area.

Irrigation

Watering a garden can be a worry; it can be tiring and tiresome. While it may be avoidable in some gardens, in some years, in some areas, most gardeners in Australia must face the task of watering come the summer. A well-mulched garden bed of soil rich in organic matter may need little additional water in a mild summer, but conditions are not always kind. Plants in pots or hanging baskets, plantings with a high water requirement in a region that cannot supply it (most lawns and backyard ferneries), vegetable gardens and, of course, greenhouses and conservatories will all need to be watered. And, of course, new plants will need frequent watering while they establish themselves in their new home. The installation of an irrigation system can make watering a painless affair.

Irrigation can be designed and installed by the home gardener with relative ease. The information that you need is simply the water flow from your garden tap, and what type of watering suits your plants best—drip irrigation, micro-spray or regular spraying. Your water flow is easily measured by timing how long it takes to fill a nine-litre bucket when your tap is on full. This information will allow you to calculate how many water lines you will need to supply the water to the outlets your garden requires. The type of outlet you require is determined by the individual plants and how you grow them. The following categories are a guide to the type of outlets available and their uses in the garden:

Pop-up systems

These have been designed for watering areas of clear lawn. The system is laid in the ground and the sprinklers sit flush with the lawn surface until the water is turned on; then, as their name implies, they pop up. Pop-up sprinklers all have a specified 'throw'—the diameter of the area they can water, given maximum water pressure—and sprinklers of various throws can be purchased to suit the needs of your lawn. The spacing of the sprinklers should allow the 'throw' of each jet to overlap that of its neighbour. The plastic, DIY systems will not stand up to an infinite amount of trampling on. If you have an area of lawn that is used for sporting activities, install sprinklers with a large throw at the corners of the area.

Dripper systems

Drip irrigation is suitable for large individual plants such as trees and shrubs, and for larger vegetables such as tomatoes, eggplants, peppers and for strawberries. Plants grown in pots or hanging baskets should be watered using drippers unless their foliage requires misting, in which case a micro-mister *on a separate line* should be used. Because drippers deliver the water directly on to the ground where it is needed, little water is lost by evaporation—compare this with a conventional sprinkler, where up to two-thirds of the water leaving the sprinkler on a hot, dry day will have evaporated before it hits the ground. Thus drippers are the most water-efficient and therefore environmentally- and budget-friendly option. Fungus-prone plants such as roses, whose foliage is best kept dry, should be watered using drippers.

Micro-spray systems

This is the best means of watering garden beds of small, dense plantings, and smaller vegetables such as carrots and lettuces. If the lines of poly-tubing are left above the ground in a vegetable garden, drippers can be easily swapped over for sprayers. This means that crop rotation can be observed with no major rearrangement of the irrigation system. Again do not mix drippers and sprayers on the same line. Container-grown plants that require misting should be watered using a micro-mister. On a hot summer's day, cool, moist shade is often what we long for, so for this reason we may choose to water plants on a pergola or around a patio by a micro-spray system. Because the throw of each jet is relatively small, evaporative losses (of water in the air) are minimised.

Within each type of irrigation system there is a choice of different water outlets; these will vary with regard to how much water they deliver and where they deliver it (near or far, full circle or only part). Some of the bigger hardware stores and nurseries and companies that manufacture irrigation systems have detailed leaflets on how to select, install and use an irrigation system. These will tell how many and what kind of water outlets you will require, what sizes and types of outlets are compatible on the same line, and how many lines you will need with the water flow rate you have from your water supply.

Installing an irrigation system usually means digging trenches to house the larger pipes. This not only looks better and is safer, it prevents the water

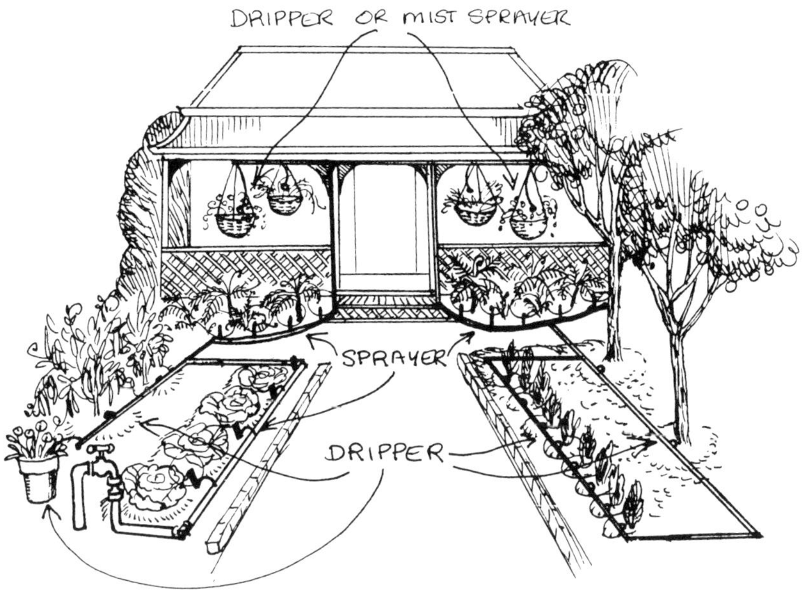

Irrigation system, showing the three types.

heating up in the sun when not in use. Within a garden bed, the tubing can be mulched over to improve its appearance if it offends, but do leave outlets clear. It is a simple affair to replace damaged tubing if necessary. It is *not* so easy to repair your gas or water lines; make sure that you know where your essential services are before you start digging. If you need to do a lot of trenching, use a narrow trenching shovel. This will make the work much lighter and means you will disrupt only a narrow strip of garden as you dig.

Any degree of automation is possible for an irrigation system, from a simple timer that will turn the water off after a set time, to a system that will water automatically for a given period at a given time interval, to a sophisticated system incorporating a sensor device that will water *only* when soil moisture levels drop below a certain point.

How often you need to water will be determined by a number of factors. These include your basic soil type, the amount of organic matter it contains and *whether or not you have mulched.* The needs of particular plants and the prevailing weather conditons will also affect the frequency with which you will need to water. Water authorities have found that many gardeners actually use more water *after* installing irrigation. It is all to easy to just turn on a system and let 'er rip—make sure that your garden really needs watering before doing so. Most plants will let you know when they need a drink long before it becomes a matter of life and death, and a thirsty plant is far easier to revive than one which has been over-watered. Take your cue from indicator plants that wilt before any others in dry conditions. I use shasta daisies for this purpose in my garden—experience will show which plants can be used in your garden for this. If still in doubt, stick your finger in the soil and see if it is wet in the root-zone region of the plants. If the soil feels moist and your plants are pert, then there is no need to water.

Frequent, shallow watering will lead to the plants developing their roots near the surface in the wetted soil; this in turn will render them far more susceptible to drying out in the heat. It is far better for all concerned—you, your water authority and of course, your plants—to water deeply but infrequently. Water moves through soils in 'fronts'—this means that water will not move to the lower levels of the soil until the top layers are thoroughly saturated, so make sure you water long enough and strong enough for this to occur. Maximise the water retention levels of your soil by mulching the beds and by increasing organic matter levels throughout.

Plants in containers will need frequent watering. How often will depend on the size of the container as well as the weather conditions and the specific needs of the plants. Plants in hanging baskets are particularly prone to drying out and should be checked daily in the heat.

The Design Process

The very first thing that needs to be done when designing a garden is to make a wish-list of all the things you would like to have if anything were possible. It may not be possible to actually have everything you put on your list, but getting them all down on paper often helps to clarify what it is you really want. Think carefully, too, about what gardening tasks you find pleasurable, and what tasks you wish to avoid. Then, armed with your wish-list, an understanding of your gardening needs and your knowledge of the possibilities of a made environment, you are ready to start designing your garden.

There is one more step to take before beginning, and that is to survey your existing garden or intended garden site and identify the problems. These will probably range from practical points (the compost bin is too far from the house, the patio too hot in summer, the slope of the path too steep), through aesthetic and 'ambience' problems (the clothesline needs screening, the north side feels too exposed, the area near the house lacks privacy), on to horticultural considerations (the roses are too crowded, the sunken lawn in drowning, the vegetable garden needs more sun). Make a list of all the points you value about the site and which you feel are serving you well, to make sure they are not overlooked later on.

Draw yourself a Site Plan. On the plan, mark in all the permanent features such as the house, the garage, the boundary fences; mark in the doors and windows. Draw it to scale as near as you can—this will help when you are trying to work out just what you can fit where later on in the process. Make it large enough to mark all the detail you will require—a scale of 1:100 is easy to work with as far as the maths goes but

1:50 gives you more drawing space. Trace or photocopy the site plan so that you have a number of copies to work with. You may already have a plan of the property from the builder or from the water authority which can be used instead, though it may be necessary to enlarge or reduce the copies to get them to a convenient size.

Let us look at the process by putting ourselves in the shoes of the imaginary gardener in the following hypothetical example: On the first of these copies of the site plan, mark in all problems and benefits of the site. Mark in the prevailing winds, problems with noise, safety and convenience, as well as the important views, and which areas are in sun and shade in high season. Mark in all the existing features including the vegetation. Identify those you wish to keep (and why), and those you wish to be rid of (ditto). This drawing is your Site Analysis.

Site analysis.

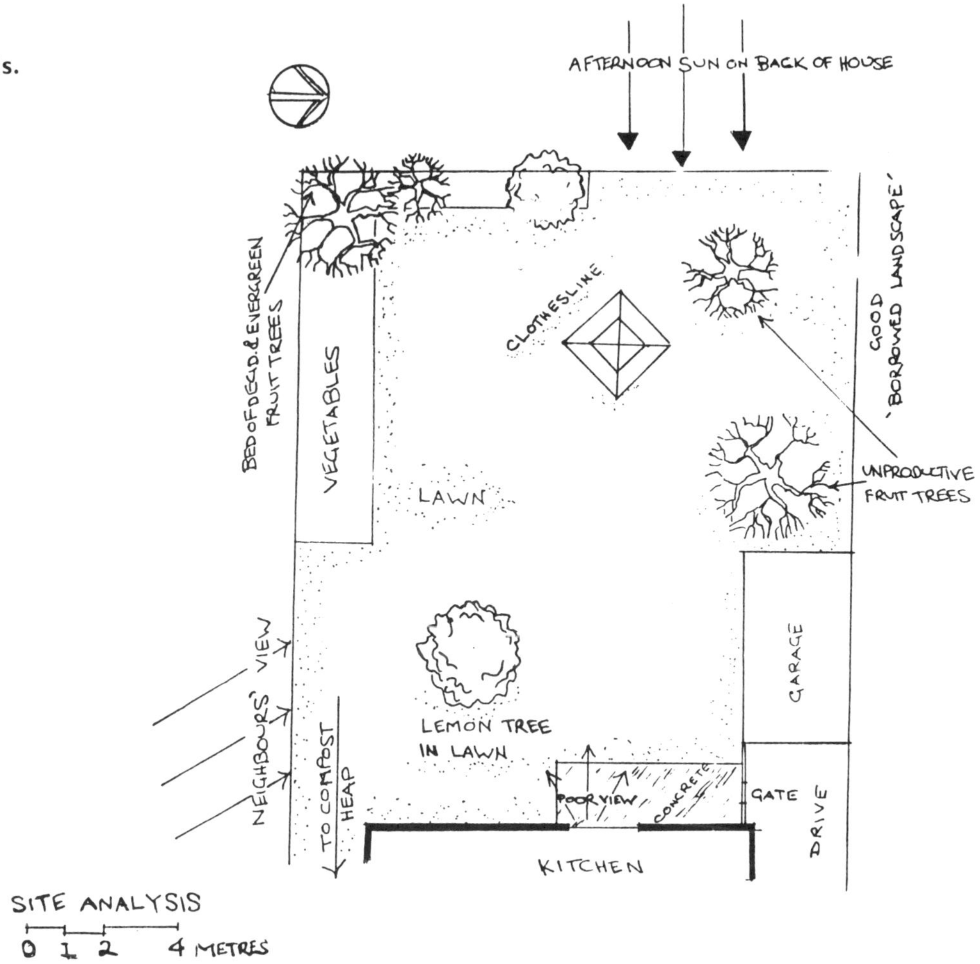

At this point, get out your wish-list and place it beside your site analysis. Remember to take into account the amount of garden maintenance that suits you best. Your wish-list may read something like this:

Wish-list

Built features
A paved entertainment area near the house, with pergola for summer shade.

Good access to conveniently located utilities areas.

A raised bed for high-maintenance vegetables.

A quiet meditation/reading area away from the house.

'Feeling' issues
A feeling of privacy throughout the garden.

A feeling of being enclosed and at peace in the quiet area.

Vegetation and wildlife
Undemanding potted plants for the paved area.

A planting of rich but restful colours in the quiet area. Low-maintenance background planting (foliage and enclosure important); flowering plants with beautiful detail and fragrance for the foreground; flowers over a long period to attract the bees; wind chimes.

Culinary herbs near the house.

At this point, see where you can solve the problems you have identified on the site *and* incorporate the items in your wish-list at the same time. For instance, in our example above, the glary, exposed area outside the back door could be shaded by a pergola then paved for use as the entertainment area. This arrangement will also minimise the distance for carrying things to and fro the kitchen. The requirement for decorative but undemanding potted plants can be combined with the desire for culinary herbs within easy reach of the kitchen. Begin to draw up a rough idea of how you might use the areas on further copies of your site plan. Do as many variations as you can think of. This will give you a Concept Plan/s. Try to visualise them in three dimensions, in all seasons and in the years to come.

When you think you are near to achieving all your important objectives in a single concept, then you can begin to draw up your final plan. This will be the plan that you will work from to calculate the materials you will need if you are doing it yourself or that you will show to the contractor if you are having the work done for you, so a reasonable amount of accuracy is desirable at this stage. You may like to show different details on separate plans for clarity's sake, say, one plan for built details and another for pots, plants, seats and ornaments. Separate construction diagrams on a larger scale will be needed for the details of any features you are building yourself. Armed with the final plan, the hard landscaping can begin. Then, once this is done, the real fun starts as the garden is planted up with the 'best and fairest' we can find.

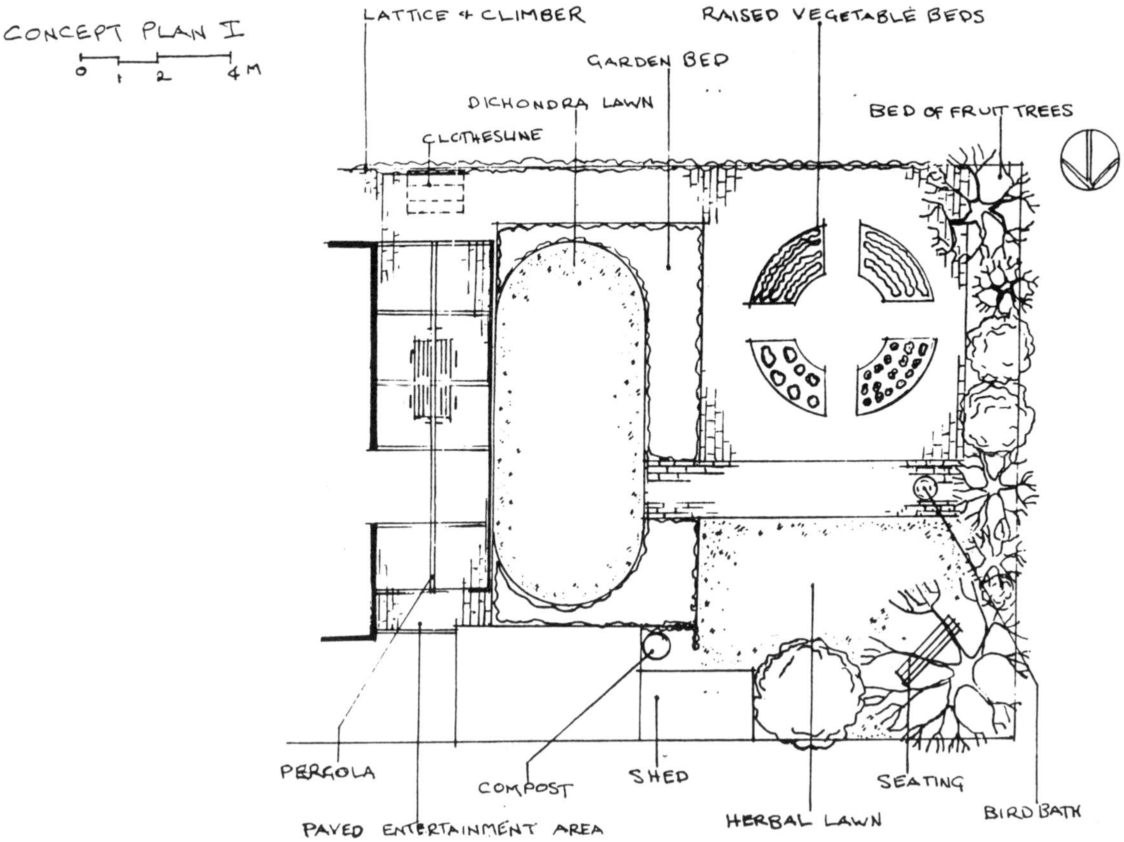

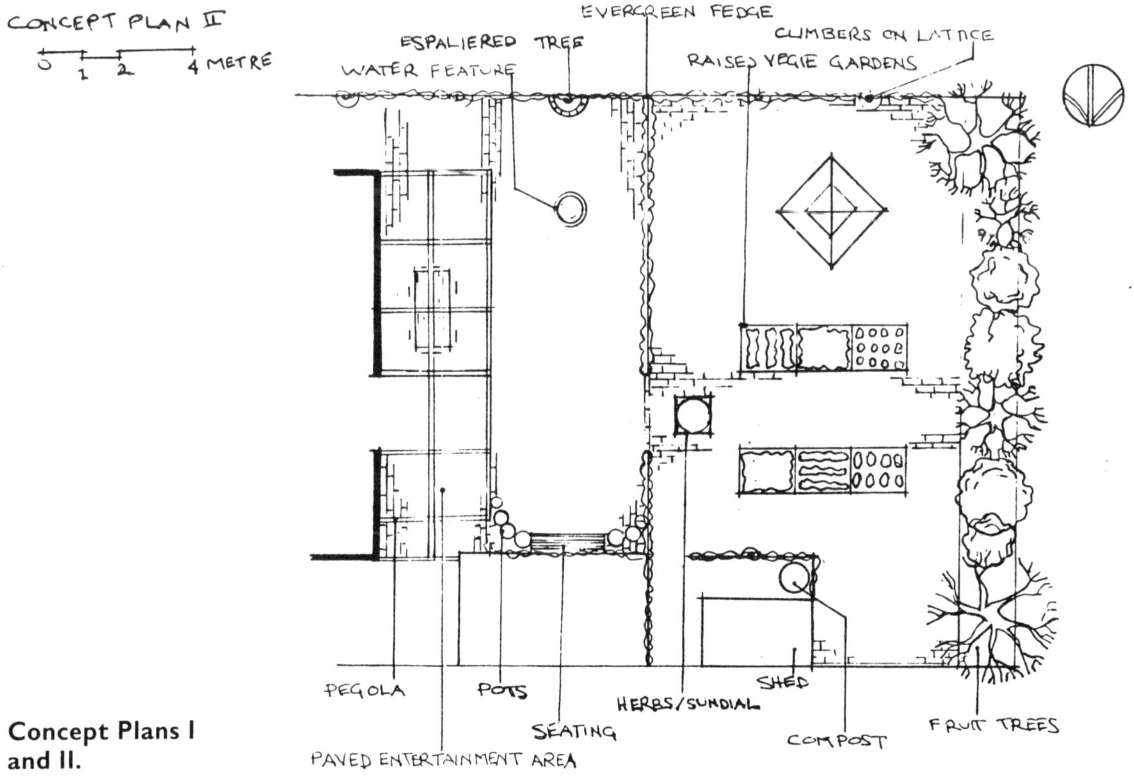

Concept Plans I and II.

6
Choosing the Right Plants

A GARDEN IS A PLACE WHERE PEOPLE AND PLANTS INTERACT, THE PLACE where our actions affect the plants, and where plants affect us, either directly, or through modifying our habitat. They affect both our physical and emotional environments. Plants may be present in our gardens to fill functional roles—to provide shade, channel the breeze, protect privacy. They may be present to provide structural roles—to form a hedge, hide the shed, frame a view. They may have a place there because of their medicinal qualities, their culinary value or their ability to ward off garden pests. Or they may be there simply because they delight!

Of course, these categories are not mutually exclusive: the wisteria covering the old shed can take our breath away with its sheer beauty, the ancient oak shading the lawn inspires a sense of reverence and awe, the nasturtiums keeping off the curly-leaf bring sunshine to our hearts. In fact, there is seldom the need to grow a plant that we find dull. The list of plants that can fill a brief is usually extensive and a plant of some charm, in accord with individual tastes, can usually be found. In any case, even the most undistinguished of old workhorses can be made lovely by a climber running through it, or a sympathetic planting at its base.

Favourites

I came upon some roses in a field.
So sweet was their fragrance
That I resolved to pick them
And take them to my loved ones.
Then their beauty caught me;
Time passed.
When next I knew myself,
All that remained of those sweet blooms
Were petals lying in the dust.

An imperfectly remembered Persian lyric poem

We most of us feel this way about something in our garden, some plant whose very beauty makes time stand still and resolve slip away. These plants are the heart and soul of a garden and we should not be without them. Sometimes it is less a plant we are in love with than a particular garden style; either way, if these plantings that so delight prove difficult, we need not abandon them, but rather, should think on restricting them to those parts of the garden where they will give us the most pleasure—a view from a window, alongside a seat—thus less will truly be more. Alternatively, we could learn to 'cheat' a little to achieve a high maintenance effect in a low maintenance way, for example, a brick border or a low wire fence could substitute for a low box hedge in a formal rose garden; a collection of pots cheerfully spilling over with plants at the edge of a paved courtyard can create a joyful, cottagy impression.

Vital to the success of any such reordering of the garden is an understanding of individual needs, regarding both the physical environment and the level of gardening activity needed to satisfy your gardening urge. It is pointless designing yourself a garden of undemanding evergreens if you start to twitch when denied a daily pottering in your plot. Nor is it sensible to have a garden that requires more of you than you care to give, though you may be physically able. Establish the level of maintenance that is right for *you*, mind, body and soul, then design the garden accordingly. As well as a list of the gardening tasks you enjoy and those you do not, you should now have a wish-list divided into:

—Layout issues
—'Feeling' issues
—Vegetation and wildlife

Practical, physical requirements—shade, a windbreak—can sometimes be met using either built structures or plants. So too with 'feeling' issues—privacy, something to screen out an ugly view, some means of making a space seem larger. Whether you select living or non-living elements to do so will depend on a number of considerations but foremost amongst these should be your preferred level of gardening activity.

Soil type will, of course, need to be considered. Large-scale modification of the soil is expensive and usually impractical. It is far better to use plants that are happy to grow in the conditions as they are, while gradually improving the soil over a period of time. Small-scale modification, for example, by raising a bed, may be a proposition, and so it may be possible to accommodate plants that are unsuited to the general soil type.

The climate, too, will impose limitations on what will grow successfully. Superimposed on the overall climate of the region will be local factors such as altitude (the higher the area, the more cold-tolerant the plants will need to be), the season of highest rainfall (wet winters similarly reduce cold tolerance), topography (do you live on the rainy side of the mountain or the dry?). As well, the microclimates in your own garden will further modify the prevailing clime and can extend the range of plants that can be grown quite considerably. For example, a north facing light-coloured brick wall will act as a heatbank and so enable you to grow frost-tender plants in a cold climate. Living in a frost-hollow where the cold air slides down a slope into your garden will mean that you will need

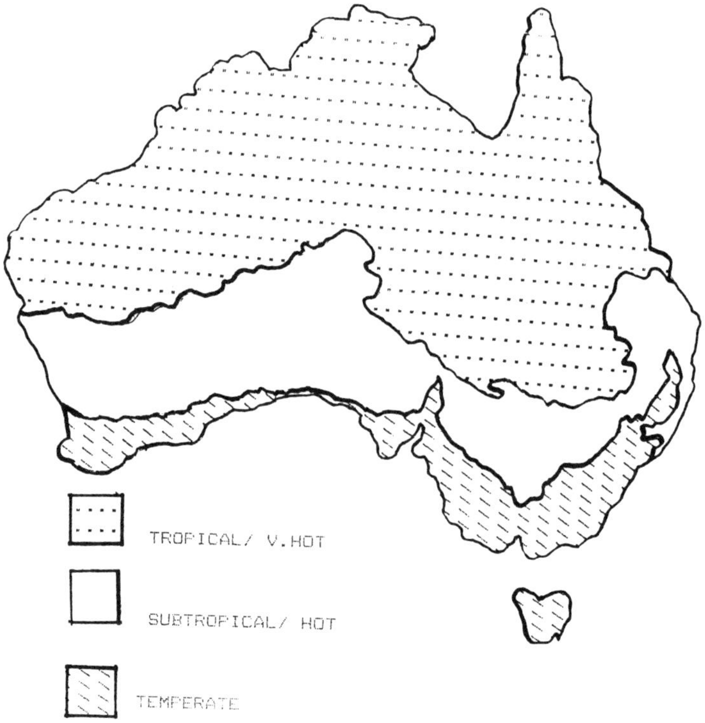

Australian climatic zones.

plants that are more cold-tolerant than those adapted to the general clime; the up-side of this is that you may well have better autumn colour than is usual in the area.

Of course, the presence of plants will also affect the microclimate. Plants may shade, break the wind, hoard the moisture, trap the frost, all of which may extend or restrict the range of plants that can be grown. In the plant lists that follow, I have given the place of origin of all the plants. Be guided by this, along with the cultural information, when deciding whether a plant is suitable for your garden, particularly if it is outside the recommended range.

I have divided the country into three climatic regions: Temperate, Subtropical and Tropical; this may be rough and ready, but fine-tuning is best left to the gardener. Unless listed as frost-sensitive, plants will tolerate cold down to —5°C (23°F). Plants listed as frost-tolerant will withstand far colder conditions than anything Australia has to offer. Many woody plants, especially trees, become more cold-tolerant as they grow; the thick layer of wood that eventually forms helps to protect them and thus they may only need protecting in the early years.

Plants for Shade

We have seen that shade is a most important garden element. If we have decided to use plants to moderate the amount of sunlight falling on the garden, we must consider whether to do so using free-standing shade trees, or by using climbing plants in combination with built structures.

This latter alternative offers a number of advantages over the former. For a start, climbers are generally fast-growing plants and will often take only two or three seasons to provide sufficient shade. In contrast, trees will take a number of years to do so, even if bought when 'advanced'. Secondly, because climbers assume, by and large, the shape of their support, they offer more design flexibility and can be accommodated in much smaller spaces. On the minus side, the cost of providing support for climbers is much higher than the cost of buying a tree, and, of course, few things have the gut-tugging effect on us of a well-grown tree. Whatever means is selected to bring shade to the garden, employ both common and aesthetic sense to your choice of shade plant.

Climbers for shade

Climbers must be amongst Nature's loveliest creations; nothing can quite take the breath away like a vast wall covered in soft leaves and beautiful, bountiful blooms; furthermore, they are also among the most useful. They come in a huge range of vigour and inclination: some billow and flow, some wend and wind; others creep and insinuate. Some climbers engulf, covering all in their path with a troubling exuberance; others, less rude, confine themselves to merely gracing their support. Some bear beautiful and fragrant flowers, some carry fruit in season. Some form a dense canopy, excluding all the light; others, somewhat lighter, provide a dappled shade.

Of greatest importance in selecting a climber is the amount of shade required, as well as when it is needed. Those living in the temperate zones, where summers are hot and the winters severe, will probably be best served by a deciduous climber that responds to the change in seasons. Those who live in the tropics are more likely to look for year-round shade, and so will opt for an evergreen cover—in any case, most normally deciduous plants are disinclined to lose their leaves when grown in tropical climes and thus are effectively evergreen.

Climbers are basically leggy plants that are unable to support themselves, and in their native habitat are to be found reaching towards the heavens through vegetation that offers them support while carrying them towards the light. Forming wood is energetically costly, and by avoiding doing so (though sometimes only in their early days), climbers are able to pour their energies into making new growth, thereby securing themselves a prime place in the ecological bun-fight.

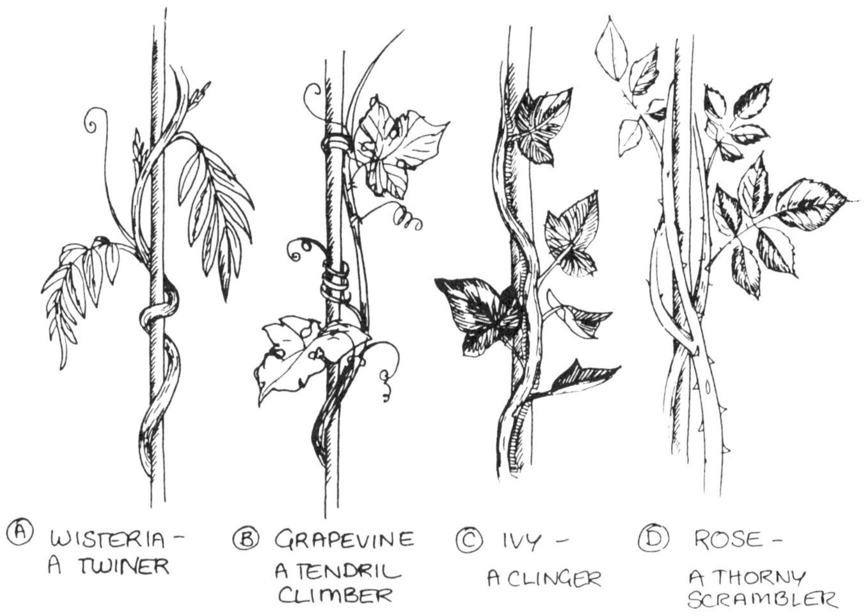

The four climber types.

Climbing plants have evolved several strategies for securing themselves to their host plants; their chosen climbing mode will influence their use in the garden. There are four main categories of climbers: Twiners, Tendril climbers, Clingers and Scramblers. Sometimes these strategies are combined. Twiners climb by twisting themselves around their support, while Tendril climbers do so by twining thread-like structures (tendrils) around the branches of their hosts. Clingers adhere to their support through suction pads or aerial roots growing from their branches and so require intimate contact between the woody tissue of the host plant and their own. Scramblers scramble their way through their hosts, catching hold by means of prickles and barbs, or by branches and leaves that grow at odd angles, or with sticky hairs or a number of other such devices.

The strategies employed by the Scramblers often render them a little antisocial and so they are perhaps the least useful category of climber from our point of view. No doubt some will dispute this, but I insist on sounding a word of caution against planting anything with thorns near any area that constitutes living space. I speak here from bitter experience—my own unreasonable prejudice in favour of the genus *Rosa* has caused me to make many an unwise decision in my time, with invariably painful consequences!

In the list of climbers that follows, plants have been selected for their dense canopy, handsome foliage, vigour and longevity. Seasonal delights are a bonus but are less important here than the everyday leaves. Almost all will be planted where much sun is received, so no shade-lovers are included. Since vigour is a prerequisite, all will require at least yearly pruning once they have grown to the desired dimensions—in a mild climate, many may well require more; all will wander into adjoining plants and properties if given half a chance. If this list seems a little spare, it is because of the rigorous selection criteria that have been applied. Only the hardiest, most reliable plants, likely to do well over the widest range of conditions of soil and climate are included. If you have your heart set on something that doesn't quite meet these standards, weigh the matter up carefully before making your final choice. Perhaps consider growing your 'fancy plant' as well as, rather than instead of, a more servicable climber. On the question of 'how many', one climber planted every 2 or 3 metres will give a dense coverage in a relatively short time. If you are prepared to wait a little longer for the desired level of shade, your less suitable 'fancy plant' could go in against every other post.

I have excluded plants that have become weeds in parts of Australia. Thus plants that might otherwise serve our purposes admirably, for example, *Thunbergia grandiflora* (Skyflower Vine)—a weed in parts of Queensland—or *Passiflora mollisima* (Banana Passionfruit)—a weed in parts of Victoria—have not been listed.

Twining climbers are perhaps better suited to pergolas than are clinging climbers. Tendril climbers usually need fine support for the tendrils to hold on to, and self-clingers are happier with something to adhere to for all but a vertical descent; however, many of the more vigorous self-clingers and tendrilous climbers could be used on a pergola if lattice, or some other form of support, is provided on the 'roof'. This will, of course, reduce the amount of sunlight that will penetrate in winter with a deciduous climber. Suitable tendril climbers and self-clingers are listed below, under 'Climbers for porches, arbours and walls' and are marked with an asterisk (*).

CLIMBERS FOR PERGOLAS

Deciduous climbers

Actinidia chinensis (Kiwi Fruit, Chinese Gooseberry) China
Subtropical and temperate zones

A robust twiner with large, dark oval leaves. The flowers are white, with a soft fragrance and appear in the spring. The brown, egg-like fruits ripen in the cooler months and are carried on the bare boughs. Both male and female plants are needed for fruiting; the plants will require a strong support. Protect from severe frosts. Full sun

Vitis species (Grape Vines) Europe; Asia
Subtropical and temperate zones

The edible grape, *Vitis vinifera* subsp. *vinifera*, has traditionally been grown both for its fruit and for the shade it provides. This tendrilous climber is an exception to the 'twiners only' rule; once a woody framework has been developed by tying in the plant as it grows, the tendrils will happily grab hold of adjacent branches. It has been trained over pergolas in many a villa in the Mediterranean since the days of the Roman Empire and can be found similarly sited in the homes of many Australian immigrants. It has much to recommend it; however, before planting one of these outside your back door, find out how fond the local wildlife is of the fruit—their presence may not be to your liking, especially if you have European wasps in your area. So-called 'ornamental grapevines' are also available. Two oriental species, *Vitis amurensis* (the Amur Vine) from China and Korea, and *Vitis coignetiae* (Crimson Glory Vine) from Japan, both have grapevine-like leaves that turn a spectacular red in the autumn. Their fruits are insignificant. All are cold-hardy, though fruiting species require summer heat to ripen the grapes. Sun

Evergreen climbers

Jasminum polyanthum (Chinese Jasmine) China
All regions

This rampant twiner soon forms a dense cover over any support that presents itself. Its white blooms are dark pink in the bud; they open in late winter and early spring and are *very* strongly scented. To some noses the perfume soon stales after the flowers open, when it becomes oppressive. Still, it is a gift to those who like it—deceptively delicate looking, this plant gives uncomplainingly of its best given half-reasonable conditions. Drought and wind resistant. Sun or semi-shade

Kennedia species Australia
Temperate regions

Both *Kennedia macrophylla* and *K. nigricans* are vigorous twiners from Western Australia. The former has handsome, fresh green leaves and carries orange-red pea flowers in the spring; the latter has ovate leaves and curious black pea flowers, again in spring time. Both species are a little frost sensitive but will tolerate dry conditions; *K. nigricans* will also tolerate wind. Sun or semi-shade

Lonicera hildebrandiana (Giant Burmese Honeysuckle) Burma
All regions

This twining climber has glossy, ovate leaves and the largest flowers of any of the honeysuckles. The creamy-white trumpet flowers age to a soft orange. They open in summertime and are sweetly scented. Although it has the potential to become enormous, *L. hildebrandiana* is easily tamed and seems content when confined to 4 or 5 metres. Protect from frosts.
Sun or semi-shade

Solanum jasminoides 'Album' (Potato Vine) South America
All regions

This plant is useful for covering large areas in a short space of time. Its terminal clusters of white 'potato' flowers are borne in summer, autumn and winter in most climates. The leaves are small and simple. Old wood often becomes bare; this is effectively counteracted by regular pruning. Will tolerate dry conditions. Sun or semi-shade

Trachelospermum jasminoides (Star Jasmine) China
Most regions

Suitable for all but the most frost-prone areas, this twiner has glossy green leaves and bears clusters of fragrant, white, star-shaped flowers in the summer. It is much faster in moist soils and is generally happier away from harsh, arid conditions. Sun through to full shade

CLIMBERS FOR PORCHES, ARBOURS AND WALLS

Here, we need not be quite so exacting in our choices. A climber will still need a reasonable amount of vigour and a good canopy, but since the area to be covered is usually smaller and the density of the support greater, we can include less vigorous climbers, as well as those that climb by means of holdfasts.

Deciduous climbers

Ampelopsis brevipedunculata (Blueberry Climber, Porcelain Grape) China and Japan
Subtropical and temperate regions

With lobed leaves like a refined grape vine, this elegant tendrilous vine is nonetheless very vigorous. In autumn it carries clusters of beautiful berries in extraordinary colours which range from dark, leaden blues through to lilac and turquoise, often in the same bunch. Good for damp sites. Protect from frosts.
*Worth a go on a pergola. Sun and semi-shade

Campsis species North America; China
Subtropical and temperate regions

Campsis radicans (American Trumpet Creeper), from North America, is a strong-growing deciduous clinger that produces aerial roots. The pinnate leaves are a glossy dark green; the orange to brick-red trumpet-flowers appear in the summer. *Campsis grandiflora* (Chinese Trumpet Vine) is very similar but has showier flowers.

*Both are possibilities for a pergola. A lattice or wire is probably not necessary. Sun

Lonicera caprifolium (Sweet Woodbine) Europe
Subtropical and temperate regions

This strong-growing twiner has naturalised in woods and hedgerows throughout much of Europe. Its creamy-yellow flowers are tinged with red and appear in the spring. They are highly fragrant, a sweet, clean fragrance that can be highly evocative.

*A possibility for a pergola if combined with lattice. Sun and semi-shade

Parthenocissus species America; Japan
Subtropical and temperate regions

Parthenocissus quinquefolia (Virginia Creeper), from Eastern North America, and *P. tricuspidata* (Boston Ivy), a Japanese species common name notwithstanding, are both clingers that use sucker discs to get a grip on their situation. Virginia Creeper has palmate green leaves (like the palm of a hand—five-leaved), while Boston Ivy has glossy, three-lobed leaves; both turn a spectacular red in the autumn. Extremely frost-hardy; *P. tricuspidata* is also wind tolerant.

*Again, these are possibilities for a pergola. Full sun to deep shade

Evergreen climbers

Akebia quinata (Five-leafed Akebia) China; Japan; Korea
Subtropical and temperate regions

This twining climber becomes semi-deciduous in colder climates. It has pretty, five-part leaves and a soft, dainty look to it. The greyish-mauve spring flowers have a gentle fragrance. Sun

Trees for shade

Trees have a powerful effect on us. Possessed of a forceful presence, a tree is a potent symbol, with mystical and religious associations that go back to before history began. There are few gardeners who would not include at least one tree in their garden for this reason alone; that they can also provide us with shade of a wonderful, quite special quality makes them perhaps the most important plants in the garden.

The majority of Australians live and garden in relatively small spaces. The once standard 'quarter acre block' has shrunk to well below one fifth of an acre, and many of us find ourselves living in ever-diminishing spaces as time goes by. The trees listed here have been selected with this 'national average' in mind. Those gardening on larger properties have a significantly wider choice of trees. For them, options include the larger oaks (*Quercus* species), elms (*Ulmus* species), and beeches (*Fagus* sp.), all of which give a wonderful shade. Or they can plant a coppice of trees which, planted singly, would provide only a light shade but which together, planted so their shadows overlap, provide good shelter from the sun. Our native eucalypts or the ever-popular silver birches can be used this way. Because they hold their leaves vertically, most cast little shadow when the sun is high.

In a very small garden such as that of a townhouse or a villa unit, shade is probably best provided by climbers. Some large shrubs such as laurestinus and even the common cotoneaster can be trained into a tree-like shape that will provide useful shade. These can be most effective *but* will need constant pruning to maintain this form. Smaller growing trees such as the ornamental plums and cherries (*Prunus* species), crab-apples (*Malus* species), and deciduous magnolias can be carefully developed by removing the lower branches from the central leader so that the branches appear above head height, otherwise their low branching patterns will make it difficult to find space underneath for more than the odd chair. They are perhaps best planted purely for their beauty. Some of the smaller Japanese maples (*Acer* species) have suitable forms but require semi-shade; they will be of no use in a sunny situation.

The trees listed here fill the following brief: they are small to medium-sized trees with a good spread and a high branching pattern; they will grow in full sun, in a wide range of soil types, provide dense shade and have a reasonable growth rate; they are relatively long-lived, and not possessed of anti-social habits such as the dropping of large limbs or squelchy fruit; they present no environmental hazard, nor do they have invasive root systems. They are well-shaped and handsome, quietly beautiful. Some have seasonal interest; all of them are green.

Good shade and a spread of at least five metres allows for living space beneath the boughs. Do not be tempted to plant a tree that you know will be too big for the spot eventually, thinking that it will be someone else's problem. You never know what lies ahead, and the headaches and heartaches that an unwise planting engenders could very well be your own.

Most of the trees listed here are available as advanced trees—these are marked with an asterisk. Planting a tree that already has several years' growth on it is an invaluable help in establishing a garden in a short time. Fast-growing but short-lived trees, such as the majority of our wattles, are recommended only as nurse trees for longer-lived species. Plant them for this purpose, by all means, but know that they will be removed after ten years or so, when your shade tree proper is of a useful size.

PREPARATION AND PLACEMENT

Care should be taken to prepare the soil properly before planting. One main reason for trees failing to thrive after planting in apparently suitable

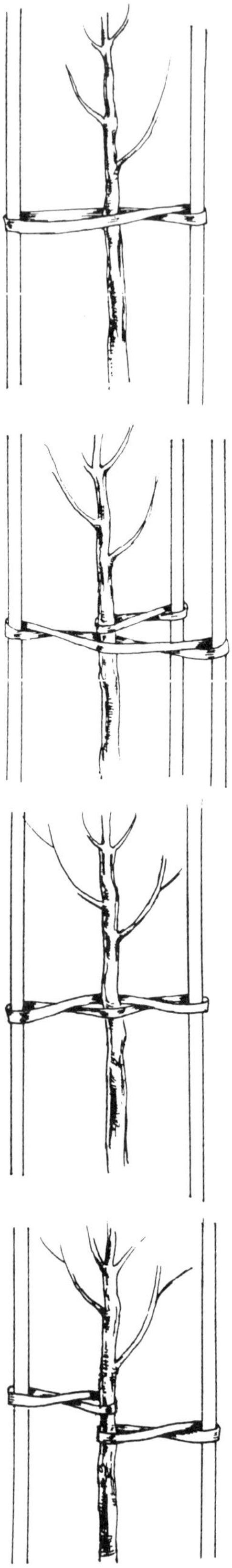

Recommended methods of supporting a tree at planting.

sites is that the physical conditions of the soil are not optimal—too porous or not porous enough. This will lead to the soil having too little water in the first case, or too little air and too much resistance for young roots in the second. This can usually be averted by proper soil preparation beforehand, however, it cannot achieve the impossible. Make sure you have selected a tree that is suited to the spot in which it is to grow—one can fly in the face of nature only so far.

Prepare a site approximately twice the size of the rootball of the tree. If possible, incorporate some organic matter into the soil several weeks in advance of the planting: partially broken down compost and some well-rotted manure is ideal. If it has not been possible to prepare the site in advance, make sure when backfilling (that is, filling the hole up after planting) that the soil is of a fine tilth. Then, top dress with a generous amount of compost and either old or pelletised manure over the entire surface of the 'hole'. There is seldom any justification for staking saplings, in fact it can prevent the development of valuable callous that would normally be formed at the base of the trunk as it flexes in the wind. With advanced trees, however, staking is necessary. They are usually top-heavy at the time of supply, so to ensure stability the tree should be secured staked, or better still, guyed. Either way, the tie/s should never be too tight, and should be checked at regular intervals for any signs of damage to the tree.

The rootball will need to be kept moist while the tree is settling in after planting. The area should be properly mulched, both to reduce water loss and to inhibit weed growth. Competition with weeds, especially the vigorous creeping grasses such as Kikuyu and Couch can have a disastrous effect on young trees.

If planting a tree to provide outdoor living space, it will most frequently be a freestanding specimen. Plant it where you intend to make use of it and, if possible, where you can appreciate its beauty from indoors. If your aim is to provide shade for your house, plant to the north, the north-west or the west of the building, depending on where the sun will hit the side of the house you wish to shade during the hottest months. Do not plant trees within 1 metre of the building.

Deciduous shade trees

**Alnus cordata* (Italian Alder) — Southern Italy and Corsica
15×8 metres (49′×26′) — Temperate and subtropical regions
A fast growing, pyramidal tree with glossy, heart-shaped leaves. The flowers are drooping catkins that precede the leaves, the fruits are little cones. This trouble-free tree is frost-hardy and will tolerate wet or compacted soils. Wind-resistant. — Sun

**Castanea sativa* (Sweet or Spanish Chestnut) — Mediterranean regions
15×12 metres (49′×39′) — Temperate regions
Worth growing for the nuts as well as the shade, this tree has long, oval,

glossy leaves with a saw-tooth edge. Flowers are pale yellow catkins in the spring. Old trees develop a spiralling, ribbed bark. Sun

**Catalpa bignonioides* (Indian Bean Tree) Southern USA
10×15 metres (33′×49′) Temperate and subtropical regions
The large, heart-shaped leaves of the Indian Bean Tree are rather like those of the Paulownia. The creamy flowers are carried in clusters and are followed by slender pods. Frost-sensitive. A golden form, **C. bignonioides 'Aureum'* is also available. Sun

**Celtis australis* (Nettle Tree) Southern Europe and the Mediterranean
12×8 metres (39′×26′) Temperate and subtropical regions
The dark-green leaves are a downy grey-green underneath. Both the foliage and the overall tree resemble that of the English Elm. The inconspicuous spring flowers are followed by brown berries which are said to be sweet. Sun

**Pyrus ussuriensis* (Manchurian Pear) Manchuria, Korea and Japan
15×10 metres (49′×33′) Temperate regions
The petals of the lovely single white blooms drift like snowflakes on the spring breezes. The glossy, oval leaves colour to a bronze-crimson in the autumn. Sun; semi-shade

**Quercus coccinea* (Scarlet Oak) Eastern North America
15×6 metres (49′×20′) Temperate and subtropical regions
The glossy, long, lobed oak leaves of this rounded tree, colour to a deep crimson in the autumn. The acorns are tiny—perhaps only 1 cm long. Will not colour well in warmer regions. Sun; semi-shade

**Tilia cordata* (Small-leafed Linden) Europe
15×10 metres (49′×33′) Temperate regions
The glossy green leaves have a grey 'bloom' underneath. The panicles of white flowers make a good show in summer. A particularly dense canopy. Sun

**Ulmus parvifolia* (Chinese Elm) China and Japan
12×15 metres (39′×49′) Temperate, subtropical and tropics
This tree has only a very short deciduous period in Australian conditions. The oval leaves are a glossy green; some trees have a pendulous form. The tree is wind and drought resistant. Sun; semi-shade

Evergreen shade trees

Agonis flexuosa (Willow Myrtle) Western Australia
10×6 metres (33′×20′) Temperate, subtropical and dry tropics
A weeping tree with willow-like leaves that are fragrant when crushed. Drought resistant, but will not tolerate waterlogged soil. Sun; semi-shade

Ceratonia siliqua (Carob Tree) Eastern Mediterranean
10×10 metres (33′×33′) Temperate and subtropical
A rounded tree with dark leathery leaves. Inconspicuous autumn flowers and edible leathery pods. Good fruiting varieties are becoming available. Drought resistant. Sun; semi-shade

**Lophostemon confertus* (Brush Box) Northern NSW, Queensland
12×6 metres (39′×20′) Temperate, subtropical and tropics
Large glossy green leaves, this rounded tree has a lovely rush of pale-green new growth in the autumn. Smooth, beige brown-marked trunk. Will tolerate compacted soils. Sun

**Magnolia grandiflora* (Evergreen Magnolia) South-eastern USA
15×10 metres (49′×33′) Temperate, subtropical and tropics
This broadly-pyramidal tree has very large glossy green leaves with a bronze underside and huge creamy-white fragrant flowers in summer. Sun; semi-shade

**Olea europea* (Common Olive) Mediterranean to India
10×8 metres (33′×26′) Temperate, subtropical and tropics
This tree is sometimes multi-stemmed in maturity, so some formative pruning may be required. The elongated, glossy green leaves are silvery underneath. The billowing foliage makes this characterful tree extremely handsome. A number of fruiting cultivars are available. Wind and drought resistant; good for seaside gardens. Do not plant where seedlings could escape into adjacent bushland. Plants are frost-hardy, but the fruits require warmth to ripen, so may not produce well in colder areas. Sun

Pinus patula (Mexican Pine) Mexico
15×10 metres (49′×33′) Temperate and subtropical
This graceful spreading conifer has layers of long fringe-like needles which hang from sweeping horizontal branches—it looks like a ballerina in a long green dress! Wind and drought resistant. Sun

Schinus molle (Peppercorn Tree) Peru
10×11 metres (33′×36′) Temperate and subtropical
This drought-resistant weeping tree is a familiar sight throughout many older parts of Australia. The silvery leaves are pinnate; the fruits are pinkish berries borne in clusters. *S. molle* will self-sow. It is dioecious—that is, there are separate male and female plants—so if you live in an environmentally sensitive area, plant only if you can obtain a male sapling. Drought resistant. Sun

**Waterhousea floribunda* (Weeping Lilly-Pilly) NSW and Southern Queensland, in coastal gullies
15×7 metres (49′×23′) Temperate, subtropical and tropics
A semi-weeping tree with glossy, luxuriant foliage. The cream flowers

are carried in early summer and are followed by white berries. Tolerant of wet soils. Sun; semi-shade

Screening With Plants

When a plant is required to cover an unsightly object or screen off an area of the garden—either to hide an ugly view, to create 'garden rooms', or to provide some privacy—an evergreen is the obvious choice. Screening is perhaps best done with climbers growing on some support, rather than free-standing trees and shrubs. Climbers have the advantage of being more or less two dimensional, and offer much quicker coverage. They also cover a structure more completely than all but a few slow growing shrubs. Any of the shrubs and trees listed later as suitable hedging plants will serve as screening. A number of the bushier, low-maintenance 'background' shrubs found further on in this chapter are also suitable. Make your selection on the basis of the size, soil and climate.

Climbers for screening

Any of the evergreen climbers listed above can be used, providing the appropriate cultural conditions can be provided. While all of the aforementioned climbers will grow in full sun, some will also grow in partial shade. Choose according to inclination, cultural conditions and the area to be covered. What follows is a list of climbers that are either less vigorous than those already listed, or else are able to grow in the shade.

Climbers (evergreen)

Ficus pumila (Creeping Fig) Japan, SE China and North Vietnam
Subtropical and temperate regions

This clinger holds on by means of aerial roots that grow from the juvenile branches. The dark green juvenile leaves are small and oval; the juvenile stems branch frequently and the climber sits neat and close to the support. The aerial roots can damage the support, so use with care. The adult growth phase is quite distinct: mature foliage is large and the mature branches grow free of the support, carrying the inedible fruit in season; this mature growth should be removed. Full sun to deep shade

Hedera helix (English or Common Ivy) Europe
Subtropical and temperate regions

Here I break with my rule of not listing any plant that is causing problems for our native flora. Ivy has become a serious weed in cool, moist parts of Tasmania, Victoria and New South Wales, so *do not* plant it if you live in an environmentally sensitive area in these parts. Outside these areas, this vigorous clinger can be a most useful garden plant. Again, it has distinct juvenile and adult phases. The juvenile leaves are lobed and the branches carry holdfast aerial roots which can damage the supporting structure. The mature leaves are larger and less lobed; the black berries are eaten by birds, who then distribute the seeds far and wide, thus the mature growth should be removed. There is a large number of selected forms available—different coloured leaves or variegations, or various leaf forms—and different degrees of vigour associated with the various selections.

Muehlenbeckia complexa (Maidenhair Creeper, Wire Vine) New Zealand
Subtropical and temperate regions
A dense but dainty twining climber with tangling, black stems and tiny, oval, dull green leaves. At its best as a 'fedge' (a climbing hedge grown on a fence—see later). Let loose amongst other vegetation, it soon becomes a terrible weed. Wind and drought tolerant. Sun to Shade

For low screening, two species of sprawling pelargoniums are excellent:

Pelargonium peltatum (Ivy-leafed Geranium) South Africa
Subtropical and temperate regions
A 'cheap and cheerful' plant, given support this leaner will reach 3 metres. The fleshy, mid-green leaves are five-lobed; the flowers bloom in terminal clusters and are borne for much of the year in warmer regions. Colour selections range from white through various pinks and reds and mauve. A form with white-variegated leaves is also available. Tolerant of dry conditions. Can also be a useful groundcover mingling between shrubs, given an annual tidy-up. Needs some frost protection. Sun

Pelargonium tomentosum (Peppermint Geranium) South Africa
3×1.5 metres (10′×5′) Subtropical and temperate regions
This sprawler has lovely, velvety lobed leaves that give off a strong peppermint scent when brushed against. Again, can be used as a groundcover between shrubs, with a yearly haircut. Unlike most pelargoniums, it needs a shaded position. Also slightly frost sensitive. Semi-shade, shade

Hedges and fedges

Hedges

A gardener may decide to plant a hedge for a variety of different reasons, such as privacy, shelter, or to make some kind of visual statement. While hedges may be either informal or formal, it is this latter type that I will be considering here. For a plant to be useful in an informal hedge, it needs only to be sufficiently dense; to be suitable for a formal hedge, rather more is demanded.

Firstly, a plant for a formal hedge must be capable of regrowing when cut back hard. Whether or not a plant has the potential to do this is simply part of its biology. Many of our native plants have this ability to resprout, evolved as a survival strategy in our bushfire ecology, and are used to great effect as formal hedging in other parts of the world with climates similar to ours. Even when possessing this potential, some plants need to have been cut back right throughout their lives in order to retain their ability to resprout. One such plant is the Monterey Cypress (*Cupressus macrocarpa*), which has been used extensively as a hedging plant throughout older settlements in Australia. Many of us will be familiar with the sorry sight of old hedges that have at some stage been neglected, then pruned hard into old wood, never to resprout again!

Secondly, a plant must grow at a rate that falls within certain limits—too slow a rate, and it will not perform its function soon enough for most of us, too fast a rate and it will need clipping more often than is sensible. Take privet, for example, which is otherwise a worthy hedging plant, but, alas, needs clipping several times a year to keep it looking neat. A clipping of once or twice a year is perhaps what we should aim for. A growth rate of around 300 mm (12″) per annum will give us a reasonable trade-off between speed of establishment and frequency of clipping.

Finally, a plant must have good, dense foliage, and leaves that are reasonably small. Since leaves can look decidedly odd and may turn brown when cut in half, a large-leafed hedge can look quite unsightly for some time after it has been clipped. The plants listed below are for medium to tall hedges; all are evergreen. A number of plants have been traditionally used in hedges for centuries, namely English Box (*Buxus sempervirens*), Yew (*Taxus baccata*) and the Holm Oak (*Quercus ilex*).

Remember that hedging plants have cultural needs which must be met. While plants of the same species will grow happily cheek-by-jowl, they resent competition from other species as much as the next plant—allow a distance of 1 metre (3′ 3″) from the base of a medium to large hedge before planting anything else. Space the hedging plants listed below 1–1.2 metres (3′ 3″–3′ 11″), with the exceptions of *Taxus baccata* (Yew) and *Quercus ilex* (the Holm Oak), which should be planted at intervals of 1.5–2.0 metres (5′–6′ 7″). Most will need regular irrigation, particularly while establishing—soaker hoses along the baseline are a good means of providing it. Do not neglect to feed hedging plants. Nutrients are required for regrowth, but in addition, there is a constant turnover of leaves in all evergreens, even though it may not be apparent. This, of course, requires energy; the foliage that is removed when a plant is clipped formed part of its energy supply and so a hedging plant must work doubly hard.

Plants for hedging

Acmena smithii (Lilly-Pilly) East Gippsland to Queensland
Temperate, subtropical and tropical

This Lilly-Pilly makes an excellent hedging plant wherever hard frosts do not prevent it being grown. I have even seen it used in some very fanciful topiary—an *A. smithii* elephant and a dinosaur are the delight of many a local, child and adult. Unclipped, *A. smithii* is a medium-sized tree, 15×7 metres (49′×23′). Sun to shade

Buxus sempervirens (English Box) Europe, N. Africa, W. Asia
Temperate and subtropical
This dense, small-leaved plant will form a cone-shaped shrub of around 3 metres (10′) if unclipped. Its dwarf form *B. s.* 'Suffruticosa' (Edging Box) is used for low formal hedging. Frost tolerant and wind resistant.
Sun to shade

Callistemon citrinus (Common Crimson Bottle Brush) Victoria, NSW and Queensland
All regions
This oft-grown callistemon is drought- and wind-resistant, tolerant of wet or compacted soils, and has fragrant, lemon-scented leaves. It still manages to flower when it is cut back hard. Unclipped, it becomes a rounded shrub of about 3 metres. Sun; semi-shade

Ilex aquifolium; *Ilex cornuta* (English Holly; Chinese or Horned Holly) Europe; China
Temperate regions
Both of these species make excellent hedging plants. English Holly is 'Christmas Holly', with spiny leaves and red berries it has many cultivars with different leaf forms and colours. If unclipped, it will become a small tree. The Horned Holly has curious glossy green leaves which bend back on themselves to give a horned effect. The autumn berries are orange. If left unclipped, it becomes a large shrub. They are both dioecious and only the female plant produces berries. Both are cold-hardy and wind resistant. Good for seaside gardens. Sun to shade

Laurus nobilis (Bay, Bay Laurel) Southern Europe
All regions
The Bay is a vigorous plant which will grow into a small tree if allowed to do so; however, it tolerates severe clipping and can even be maintained as a standard. Its fragrant dull-green leaves are used in cooking when dried. It is wind and drought tolerant. Sun; semi-shade

Photinia species Asia
Temperate, subtropical
There is a number of species of photinia that are excellent as hedges. These include *Photinia serrulata* (Chinese Hawthorn), *P. glabra* 'Rubens' (Red-leafed Photinia) from China and Japan, and the Sydney-raised *P.* ×*fraseri* 'Robusta'. The first of these species is tolerant of wind and salt and will grow into a small tree if unclipped; the last two would make large shrubs. The two shrubby plants both have red new growth which ages to green; clipping induces a flush of new red growth. They all carry trusses of clear white flowers in the spring. Sun; semi-shade

Quercus ilex (Holm Oak) Mediterranean
Temperate, subtropical
The Holm Oak has long been used in Europe as a hedging plant. It has

very dark, glossy leaves and small acorns. Unclipped it will in time become a large tree (20×15 metres) (66′×49′). Wind- and drought-resistant. Good for seaside gardens. Sun; semi-shade

Taxus baccata (Yew) Europe, Asia Minor, North Africa
Temperate, subtropical

The Yew makes a superb hedge; unclipped, it will become a large tree. There are many cultivars of the plant available, but the species itself is the best suited to hedging. Very cold tolerant. Toxic to stock.
Sun; semi-shade

Fedges

Fedges are simply hedges formed by growing a climber over a structure, usually wire fencing. They really offer the best of both worlds—like fences, they are fast and narrow; like hedges, they are green, beautiful and offer habitats to local wildlife. For a wire fedge, all of the dense-growing evergreen twiners and tendril climbers already recommended for pergolas, screening and arbours are suitable, particularly *Akebia quinata*, *Muehlenbeckia complexa* and *Trachelospermum jasminoides*, all of which grow better and bushier when given a regular trim. If you have a solid support structure, select an evergreen self-clinger to suit your conditions, such as Common Ivy (*Hedera* species) or Creeping Fig (*Ficus pumila*).

Other plants for fedges

Clystostoma callistegioides (Argentine Trumpet Vine) South Brazil, Argentina
Temperate, subtropical

This tendril climber has glossy, pinnate leaves; the mauve, funnel-shaped flowers are carried in the spring and early summer. The pods which follow are prickly, so clip *soon after flowering*. Protect from frosts.
Sun; semi-shade

Distictus buccinatoria (Mexican Blood Flower) Mexico
Temperate, subtropical, tropical

This tendril climber has attractive pinnate leaves with oval leaflets; the crimson trumpet flowers bloom throughout the summer. Cold-sensitive, but will grow in the warmer temperate regions if given some frost protection. Sun

Background Planting: Some Undemanding Shrubs and Groundcovers

If you have decided to 'rationalise' your garden—and to restrict your demanding but much loved favourites to just a few key places, you may find yourself with empty spots in need of filling, and no clear idea of what to use for this. The following is a brief list of low-labour shrubs—some almost qualify as small trees—that, for most of the season, are content to remain in the background.

Evergreen shrubs

Abelia × grandiflora (Glossy Abelia) Hybrid of garden origin
2 × 2.5 metres Temperate, subtropical
This dense shrub has small dark-green bronze-tinged leaves and an airy texture. Its arching branches carry terminal clusters of small white or pale-pink trumpet-flowers throughout much of the hot weather. Each flower is held in a russet-brown calyx which persists after the petals have dropped. Frost tolerant. Sun; semi-shade

Escallonia species South America
All regions
Escallonias generally are useful, fast-growing shrubs that originate (or are hybrids or selected forms of species that originate) in temperate South America. *Escallonia rubra* var. *macrantha* (Common Escallonia) (3 × 2 metres/ 10′ × 6′ 6″), and *E. bifida* (4.5 × 3 metres/15′ × 10′) are both bushy evergreens with deep green glossy leaves and clusters of small, simple flowers. The first species has rose-pink blooms, the second has white. Drought tolerant and tolerant of salt-laden winds, these species are good screening plants in coastal areas. Sun

Eriostemon myoporoides (Long-leaf Waxflower) Victoria, NSW
2.5 × 2.5 metres (8′ 2″ × 8′ 2″) All regions
This lovely native forms a rounded shrub which carries its pink-tinged white flowers over spring and early summer. Usually found sheltered by taller plants in its natural habitat, it blooms well in sun or semi-shade. Protect from severe frosts. Sun, semi-shade

Hakea laurina (Pincushion Hakea) Western Australia
5 × 3 metres (16′ 5″ × 9′ 10″) Temperate regions
The Pincushion Hakea has grey-green, Bay Laurel-like leaves, and usually pink pom-pom flowers in winter and spring which attract the birds. Drought tolerant. Sun

Juniperus chinensis 'Pfitzeriana' Garden-raised
1 × 3 metres (3′ 4″ × 9′ 10″) Temperate and subtropical
A lovely, 'whooshy' little conifer with arching branches and grey-green foliage. Tolerant of wind, drought, and salt spray. Sun to shade

Melaleuca species Australia

M. amallaris (Bracelet Honey Myrtle) Victoria, NSW and Queensland
5 × 7 metres (16′ 5″ × 23′) Temperate and subtropical
This is fast growing, with small, needle-like leaves which give a filmy

effect, though with a less interesting texture. High wind and drought resistance; tolerant of wet or compacted soils. It is fast-growing but short-lived, so plan to replace. Sun

M. decussata (Totem Poles) South Australia and Victoria
2×2.5 metres (6′ 6″×8′ 2″) Temperate
The leaves are grey-green, narrow and oblong. The flowers are small pale-mauve bottlebrushes and are carried over spring and summer. The woody seed capsules give the plant its common name. High tolerance of compacted or waterlogged soils. Good wind and salt tolerance.
Sun and semi-shade

M. huegelii (Chenille Honey Myrtle) Western Australia
4×1.5 metres (13′×5′) Temperate and subtropical
This graceful, open-growing shrub has a diffuse but almost velvety texture, with creamy flowers which are carried in great numbers in the spring. Sun and semi-shade

M. quinquenervia (Broad-leafed Paper Bark) Queensland
10×5 metres (33′×6′ 6″) All regions
This native of Queensland's swampy coastal regions is a small tree rather than a shrub but is included here for its sheer adaptability: it is wind and drought tolerant, tolerant of compacted or waterlogged soils and of salty sea spray. It is, however, a little frost sensitive. It has larger flowers and foliage than these other melaleucas and so does not have their wispy look. The white bottlebrush flowers are bird-attractants. Sun

Pittosporum species

Pittosporum eugenoides (Tarata) New Zealand
8×4 metres (26′×13′) All regions
This plant is a small tree, though this may come as a surprise to those used to seeing it as a clipped hedge or a container-grown bush. The leaves are light green with wavy margins. The cream-variegated form *P. e.* 'Variegatum' (Silver Tarata) is very popular as a container plant in shopping centres. Tolerates wind, drought, and all manner of insult!
Sun; semi-shade

P. tenuifolium (Kohuhu) New Zealand
6×3 metres (20′×10′) Temperate and subtropical
This graceful tree has light green leaves with wavy margins; both the bark and the night-fragrant flowers are black. This species has given rise to many popular cultivars including the small leaved 'James Stirling', the purple-leaved 'Purpureum', the smaller growing 'Irene Watson' which has leaves marbled with cream, and the diminutive 'Tom Thumb'. Wind resistant. Sun; semi-shade

Plumbago auriculata (Plumbago) South Africa
1×3 metres (3′×10′) All regions
The indolent Plumbago is a sprawling shrub with light green leaves; the pale blue starry flowers are produced over a long period in summer and autumn; a white form, *P. a.* 'Alba' is also available. Drought and wind tolerant; good for seaside plantings. Sun

Raphiolepsis umbellata (Yeddo Hawthorn) Japan
1.5×2 metres (4′ 10″×6′ 7″) Temperate and subtropical
A dense dome-shaped shrub with dark green leathery leaves and panicles of fragrant white flowers in the spring. Wind and drought tolerant, and generally as tough as old boots, but slow growing. Sun to shade

Sparmannia africana (African Hemp) South Africa
3×3 metres (9′ 10″×9′ 10″) All regions
This fast-growing, formless and rather bulky shrub has large, fresh green maple-like leaves; the white pom-pom flowers are produced for most of the year. A double-flowered form *S. a.* 'Flore Pleno' is also available.
Sun; semi-shade.

Viburnum tinus (Laurustinus) Mediterranean
3×2 metres (9′ 10″×6′ 7″) All regions
This is a dense upright rounded shrub. It flowers all winter, the white blooms opening from brownish-pink buds. Wind and drought resistant; good for seaside gardens. Will take severe clipping. Sun; semi-shade

Westringia fruticosa (Coastal Rosemary) Coastal NSW
2×4 metres (6′ 7″×14′) Temperate and subtropical
The small, spiky leaves resemble herbal Rosemary, hence the common name. The flowers, too, are similar in form, and may be anything from white through to mauve. Can be clipped. Wind and drought resistant; salt tolerant. Sun

Deciduous shrubs

If you would like some autumn colour, these shrubs put on a good show without giving you hours of work clearing the fallen leaves, as perhaps would a larger plant.

Berberis thunbergii (Barberry) Japan
1.5×1.5 metres (5′×5′) Temperate
This bush has tiny leaves and an arching habit. The spring flowers are small and yellow, the berries scarlet. In autumn, the leaves turn a splendid crimson. The purple-leaved form, *B. t.* 'Atropurpurea' is often grown. Can be clipped, but its cascading form is most attractive. Its dense and spiny growth provides protection for small birds. Cold tolerant. Sun

Cotinus coggygria (Smoke Bush) SE Europe and the Mediterranean
3×4 metres (10′×13′) Temperate
The Smoke Bush has paddle-shaped leaves that turn a wonderful burnt orange in autumn. Hazy plumes of smoky brown flowers are produced in the spring. Two purple-leaved forms are available: 'Royal Purple' and the more bronze-toned 'Foliis Purpureis'. Frost tolerant. Sun; semi-shade

Viburnum opulus (Guelder Rose) Europe, North Africa, Northern Asia
3×2 metres (10′×6′ 6″) Temperate
The lobed, maple-like leaves turn a rich red in the autumn, with white ball-like clusters of flowers in spring, followed by red autumn berries. Found in moist valleys, it has a high tolerance of compacted soils and waterlogging. The cultivar 'Sterile', the Snowball Bush, with large, white, pom-pom flower clusters, is more commonly grown than the species; it is sterile, and carries no berries. Full sun to shade

Groundcovers

A groundcover is a plant which grows in such a way that its foliage forms a dense cover over the soil. They are used as an attractive way of filling a relatively large space in a garden in an undemanding, trouble-free way while inhibiting weed growth in that space at the same time. Many of us grow a number of pretty mat-forming small plants in the foregrounds of our gardens, mostly for their flowers but sometimes for their foliage. Usually they will require some form of regular, seasonal maintenance—cutting back after flowering (*Anthemis tinctoria*, Ox-eye Chamomile), weeding from lawns or adjoining beds (*Ajuga repens*, Bugle), cutting back from paths over which they have strayed (*Convolvulus maritima*), or the removal of volunteer seedlings (*Erigeron karvinskianus*, Mexican Daisy). The list I have compiled below is of plants which need virtually no seasonal care and require thinning or cutting back only every year or two at the most.

Most of us think of low growing plants when the term 'groundcover' is used, but taller plants can do the job just as well; the height of the plant chosen as a groundcover will depend on how and where it is to be used and is generally a design decision rather than one based on practical considerations. For a plant to function well as a groundcover it must:

- Form a persistently dense mat of leaves
- Be long-lived and easily renewable
- Be trouble-free under the conditions of the site
- Not stray unduly beyond its allotted space. To do so will result in the plant being any or all of the following: dangerous/unsightly/requiring a high degree of maintenance.

A groundcover may be a clump-forming plant, a stoloniferous plant (that is, a plant which spreads by horizontal runners that root and shoot as they go), or a prostrate shrub. All may give effective low-maintenance cover for an area. Climbers may also be used as groundcovers but will often require more work, for they are wont to get ideas above their station and wander high and low.

Before planting, make sure you give some thought to the following:

— Planting more than one species of groundcover will usually result in one species out-growing the other. It is safer to plant areas out with just one single species.

— Space plants so that they will join up to form an effective cover in a reasonable length of time. This will mean planting at considerably less than the mature width of the plant when grown as an individual specimen. Plants of the same species do not usually compete with one another—just think of the 'mass plantings' in natural plant communities—thus they can be planted at very close spacings with no ill effect. I would suggest you plant them at intervals of one-quarter to one-third of their predicted width at five years (see below).

— Mulch between the plants at planting time to keep the weeds down until such time as individual plants fuse together to give effective cover.

— Groundcover plants are still *plants* and will require some degree of care, including watering during a dry spell in some cases. They cannot be expected to look their best (or do their job) if grown in a situation to which they are not suited.

— Groundcovers may be an expensive option if the plants have to be purchased. If the area concerned is seldom seen, mulching may be a better option; it will definitely be a cheaper one.

Plants for groundcover

Below is a list of low-maintenance, hard-working, effective, evergreen groundcovers. Their size five years after planting from vigorous tube stock is given, rather than their mature size, as this is a better guide to the spacing required for cover in a reasonable (by the gardener's definition) time. (Other plant descriptions give the 'average' size of the mature plant.)

Ajuga 'Jungle Beauty' — Garden origin
150 × 450 mm (6″ × 18″) — All regions
This groundcover spreads by means of stolons, and has bold, club-shaped leaves, often with a purple-bronze margin; it carries low spikes of dark blue flowers in the spring. High tolerance of waterlogging. Frost tolerant.
Sun to shade

Arundaria viridistriata (Dwarf Goldstripe Bamboo) Japan
750 mm × 1 metre (2′ 6″ × 3′ 3″) Temperate and subtropical
This vivid gold-striped dwarf bamboo will stray though not with the vigour of many bamboos. Still, its usefulness as a low-maintenance groundcover is restricted to areas bounded by hard surface. Good for lightening up a dark corner or a shaded courtyard. Sun, semi-shade

Coprosma acerosa (Sanddune Coprosma) New Zealand
75 mm × 1.5 metres (3″ × 5′) Temperate and subtropical
This is a dense, prostrate shrub with narrow darkgreen leaves. The plant is dioecious (separate male and female plants) with pale-blue berries on the female in the autumn. If you want berries, go for one male plant, the rest female; if not, go for all male. Use plants propagated vegetatively from the same stock. Sun

Grevillia species

Grevillea montis-cole (Mount Cole Grevillea) is a dense, low-growing shrub, 300 mm × 1.5 m (1′ × 5′) with holly-like leaves, including the prickles, and red toothbrush flowers in winter; from central Victoria, it is frost-hardy and can be grown in either full sun or semi-shade. The Western Australian *G. thelmanniana* (Spider Net Grevillea) has soft rosemary-like leaves and red flowers. This prostrate shrub (150 mm × 1 metre) has both grey and green leaved forms; the green leaved form is denser growing and is a far better groundcover. Drought tolerant, it requires full sun. Both plants are wind resistant and are suitable for temperate and subtropical regions.

Hypericum calycinum (Rose of Sharon) SE Europe, Western Asia
250 × 600 mm (10″ × 2′) Temperate and subtropical
This is a creeping shrubby plant that spreads by means of stolons. It has oval green leaves and buttercup-like yellow flowers with beautiful stamens produced over the summer. It will grow in full sun but is happier—and a thicker groundcover—in the shade. High tolerance of wind, drought, and compacted soils. Sun to shade

Juniperus species

Juniperus horizontalis (Creeping Juniper) Eastern North America
50 mm × 1 metre (2″ × 3′ 3″) Temperate
This prostrate conifer has fan-like branches and green or blue-green foliage. It creeps by the branches rooting as they go. It is an excellent groundcover, though very slow growing. Drought and cold tolerant.
Sun; semi-shade

J. conferta (Shore Juniper) Japan
200 mm × 1 metre (8″ × 3′ 3″) Temperate
This prostrate shrub has fresh-green foliage. It requires excellent drainage—it is susceptible to infection by *Phytophthera* (a fungal rot currently claiming some of our native forests) when planted in damp sites. High drought and wind resistance; frost tolerant; good for seaside gardens. Sun

Myoporum parvifolium (Creeping Myoporum) Southern Australia
60 mm × 1.5 metres (2.5″ × 5′) Temperate regions
This dense prostrate shrub roots as it goes. The small white summer flowers nestle amongst the blunt, narrow leaves. High tolerance of wind and drought; useful for seaside plantings. Sun; semi-shade

Container-Grown Plants

There are clear advantages to growing plants in containers. First and foremost, containers allow you to grow plants where plants simply could not be otherwise grown. Pots on a balcony, window boxes, hanging baskets allow us to carry Nature into places otherwise bare of her influence; light-weight pots can be moved around to display seasonal features, or just for the sake of a change. Containers allow us to grow plants that are unsuited to the conditions that prevail in the area without an enormous imput of energy and resources—by using the appropriate growing medium and supplying the requisite care, plants from an arid region can be grown in a high rainfall area, phosphate-sensitive plants grown in an area treated with superphosphate, frost-tender plants protected from the cold.

Finally, as a design element, a container can bring a plant into sharp focus, providing far more visual impact than would otherwise be the case. And the pots themselves can introduce a further decorative element, for the choice these days is vast. Whether your taste turns to traditional terracotta, ornate Victoriana, or post-modern mosaics, there are pots, bold and bright for strong stylistic statements, or quiet and classic, to harmonise and blend.

There are, of course, disadvantages to pots. First and foremost amongst these is the amount of care that container-grown plants require. The roots of a plant within a pot can look no further for water and precious nutrients than the container in which it stands. A container-grown plant may easily dry out and can quickly run out of essential minerals and it falls to the gardener to supply the plant with these requirements. And, because the growing medium in a pot is without the insulating effects of the garden soil, roots are more likely to freeze or to fry in extremes of temperature.

Pests and diseases are always more of a problem with container-grown plants; if you wish to avoid spraying every other week, then either a good deal of effort must be put into selecting plants that are trouble-free when pot-grown, or you must resign yourself both to picking off infested plant parts as soon as they appear and to the possibility of unhappy looking plants. I would suggest that the former approach is generally more satisfactory, and certainly less heartbreaking.

Stability, too, is a concern with larger plants, and must be supplied by a container of suitable weight; top-heavy pots can topple in a breeze, sometimes losing their contents with disastrous consequences. Where possible, plants should be developed by formative pruning into a roughly pyramidal form with a central leader: most container-grown fruit trees and dense-growing shrubs are candidates for this treatment. When a spreading form is a feature of the plant, for example with the many graceful cultivars of the Japanese Maple, then a wide and weighty pot will best display its graces *and* keep it upright in a wind.

The only limits to what you can grow in containers are the space you can offer the roots and the stability you can provide to the plant. In the appropriate pot, with the appropriate care, plants from every category can be grown—trees, shrubs, bushes, bulbs, natives, exotics, herbacious perennials, annuals, vegetables, herbs, standards, climbers, cacti and succulents, and even water-plants.

Container size

There are two main points to consider when selecting the size of your pot. The first of these is the size of the plant to be grown. It is preferable to use a container that will allow a reasonable amount of root growth. It is said that plants do not grow well in pots that are much too big for them. I have never put this to the test but I can find no logical reason why plants should be made unhappy by having an abundance of space in which to spread their roots. The larger the pot, the less likely the plant is to run out of water and nutrients, or for the roots to overheat or be frost-bitten. Certainly, though, it can look a little odd to have a tiny little plant in a great big pot; the situation is easily remedied by massing fast-growing annuals in the empty space—especially useful in the case of young trees and shrubs in temporarily over-large containers.

The second point to consider is the weight of the pot, particularly if you will want to move the plant around. Larger containers can become very heavy when filled with potting mix; this can make repotting difficult, and moving them nigh on impossible. Casters or plant trolleys can be used under the containers so they can be easily moved.

Potting mix

Plants grown in containers are susceptible to both drying out and to overwatering. Drowning is one of the most common causes of death of plants in containers; a drowning plant will usually signal its plight by confusingly behaving rather as if it has some form of deficiency; its leaves turn yellow, then finally drop. By the time things get to this stage, the situation is often irreversible, even if the cause of the plant's distress is recognised and the roots are allowed to dry out.

It is recommended that you use a potting mix that has been formulated for use in a container. A commercially prepared mix from a reliable manufacturer will be the safest and the easiest; it should retain some water yet be free-draining, contain sufficient nutrients to last the plant for some time, and allow easy passage to the roots as they grow through. Of course, it can be quite expensive to use such a mix if you have a number of containers to fill, and the temptation to use garden soil may be great. But most garden soils will not drain fast enough for use in containers and will require the addition of a gritty material such as coarse sand; by the time the soil has been diluted down with the grit it will also need additional nutrients. In some cases, water-retentive material such as peat or vermiculite will need to be added; the pH may also need to be adjusted. It is usually neither cheaper nor more convenient to go through all this.

It may seem a peculiar piece of doublespeak that you are told that pots dry out more readily than a garden bed, but that drainage can also be more of a problem. This is because of the way that water moves through a growing medium, be it potting mix or soil. Water moves through under the effects of gravity but it is also pulled through a medium by the capillary action of the fine pores (see Chapter 4 under 'Soil Structure'). When the water reaches the bottom of a pot, this suction effect of the medium abruptly runs out, with a consequent wet layer of medium in the bottom of the pot. This wet layer at the base can lead to waterlogging with the plant roots suffocating or even rotting. Potting mixes are designed to avoid this pooling in the base.

Those who are growing food crops in containers may have a further concern about their potting mix. If they are attempting to 'grow organic' they will probably prefer to 'roll their own'. A suitable mix can be obtained by combining:

1 part (by volume) garden soil
1 part well-rotted compost or peat moss
1 part coarse washed sand

If concerned, check the pH of the mixture—most vegetables grow best in a neutral pH (6.0–7.0), although a few have a preference for either higher or lower values, for example, beetroot will crop better in slightly alkaline (lime) conditions. If too low, add Dolomite at the rate recommended by the manufacturer; if too high, wood ash can be used to lower it, although the amount needed will vary with the ash and will need to be determined by trial and error. If planting annuals, be they food crops or flowering plants, add a slow-release fertiliser such as pelletised manure at the time of planting; top dress with organic fertilisers as needed as you would for plants in the ground.

Soil that contains pests or diseases should not be used as a growing medium; however, it is possible to pasteurise soil so that most pests and pathogens are destroyed while the majority of beneficial organisms remain. Commercially, this is done by blowing air and steam through moist soil and then holding the temperature of the soil between 60 and 80°C (140 and 176°F) for 30 minutes. This is difficult without special equipment. Microwave ovens *can* be used to pasteurise the soil; heat the soil to 70–80°C (158–176°F), then wrap it up and store it so that it stays at over 60°C (140°F) for 30 minutes. Obviously, only a small amount of soil can be pasteurised this way at any one time.

If growing larger plants in containers, choose a potting mix that is sufficiently heavy to provide good anchorage; mixtures containing perlite or vermiculite will probably not be sufficiently heavy.

To crock or not to crock

Crocking is the use of a layer of broken pottery or coarse gravel in the bottom of a plant container. There are many gardeners who swear by crocking as the key to successful container culture. There is no clear reason why this should be so; in fact, many experts completely dismiss the idea. The coarse material at the bottom has no more 'pulling-power' than the open air below the pot and should not, on the face of it, improve drainage at all. Indeed, in certain circles, crocking is felt to make matters worse by taking up space that would be better filled with well-draining potting mix in which the roots of the plant could grow. Personally, I think it highly likely that the drainage holes of the containers are more prone to blocking than is often recognised, particularly if soils or 'fines' are used in the potting mix; the layer of open material at the bottom may then make a critical difference to the drainage. To be on the safe side, make periodic checks to see that your pots are draining as they should.

Watering and feeding

Container-grown plants are dependent upon the contents of the pot to supply their needs for water and nutrients. Most of us will have seen the sad sight of roots protruding from the drainage holes of a pot, hungrily searching for whatever it is they lack. The needs of the plant must be met almost entirely by the gardener. Watering a large number of pots by hand is something not all gardeners find pleasurable, and it may be preferable to put in an irrigation system to deal with it. This can be especially useful with large pots, or pots that are hard to reach (see Chapter 5). It is especially important to keep up the water with food crops, particularly fruit trees—it takes up to one thousand litres of water to produce one kilogram of fruit! However, do be sure that your plant actually needs watering before doing so—stick your finger in the potting mix and *feel* it if you are uncertain.

Plants under cover, for example on a porch or a balcony sheltered from the rain may receive no overhead watering. Their leaves will need rinsing from time to time to remove accumulated grime and sometimes insects.

Plants growing in containers will soon exhaust the supply of nutrients in the potting and will need regular feeding. This is best done using a slow-release fertiliser. There are a number of these granulated plant foods on the market now. Those wishing to grow organically can use 'Blood and Bone', pelletised manure or a seaweed extract. Choose one which has been deodorised—you will regret it if you don't; in a small space, there is no escaping strong smells, and, believe me, some seaweed extracts smell like something washed up by the tide then left to moulder in the summer heat! Be ever-vigilant for signs of mineral deficiency, and feed the plant as soon as any signs are detected.

Plant selections

Vegetables

Those of us growing vegetables in pots will almost always be doing so because of space restrictions, thus it makes sense to use bush forms of vegetables where these are available, rather than the more usual sprawling or climbing forms unless you have some vertical space to accommodate them. Bush forms of beans, cucumbers, pumpkin and zucchini are now available. Tomatoes are frequently grown in containers; often they will need staking, although non-staking varieties are available. Glancing through a book recently, I saw a photograph of a small-growing cherry tomato plant in full fruit, trailing over the sides of the hanging basket in which it was growing. It looked both decorative and delicious and is something which definitely warrants investigation. The miniature small fruiting varieties Tiny Tim should be suitable.

Some naturally bushy vegetables, such as eggplant and capsicum, do very well in pots, as do crops that grow new leaves, such as rhubarb, silverbeet, Chinese cabbage and small-headed European cabbages; culinary herbs and salad greens—lettuce, endive, nasturtiums—are very successful in containers. Potatoes can be grown in large pots, or in a pile of old tyres. Some vegetables require a deeper root run than we can usually give them in containers: vegetables such as cauliflowers and broccoli, and the longer root crops, such as carrots. These are generally best left to those with garden beds; however, plant breeders have realised that there is a market for vegetables that can be grown in small spaces. New varieties are coming on the market all the time, so check the seedling racks and displays of seed packets before giving up on a particular vegetable.

Fruit trees

Apple trees on dwarfing rootstock (see Chapter 4) are suitable as container-grown plants. So, too, is the new compact-column variety, 'Ballerina', although it does not carry much fruit. The quince is a small, neat tree and could also be grown in a pot, as can the medlar.

Peaches and nectarines are tip or lateral bearers so a good deal of new wood must be left on to ripen each season. This makes it difficult to keep them trained in a compact stable shape; only the genetic dwarf peach and nectarine lend themselves easily to pot culture. If, however, you have wall space available to grow full-sized trees against, they are a possibility.

Wall space makes it possible to grow grape vines and passionfruits in pots as well. It also makes the long-caned berry fruits, such raspberries and the blackberry family a proposition—that is, blackberries, loganberries, boysenberries and others; in fact, growing this group in pots prevents the plants from spreading by horizontal roots. Watch the prickles though! Gooseberries and black and red currants can also be grown in containers.

In northern European countries during Victorian times, orangeries were all the go with the gentry. Orange trees grown in large pots were set outside in the summer, then brought indoors to overwinter in the greenhouse or conservatory. In our somewhat milder climate, orange and grapefruit trees are vigorous plants and require large containers. More easily accommodated are other members of the citrus family, such as lemons, mandarins, cumquats and limes. Seek local advice about the variety suited to your area.

Fig trees, feijoas, cherry guavas and pomegranates can also be grown in pots; these last three are often grown as ornamentals and make interesting and attractive pot specimens.

Tropical fruit trees are large, vigorous plants unsuitable for growing in containers, with the exception of pineapples. Bush varieties of melons are a possibility in parts of Australia where climate and space permit—a very large pot is needed.

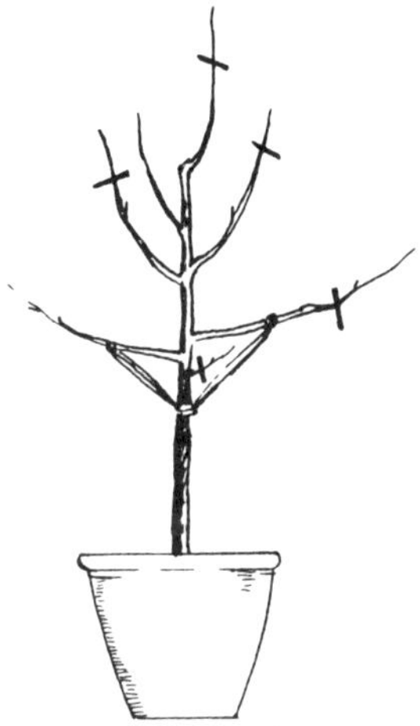

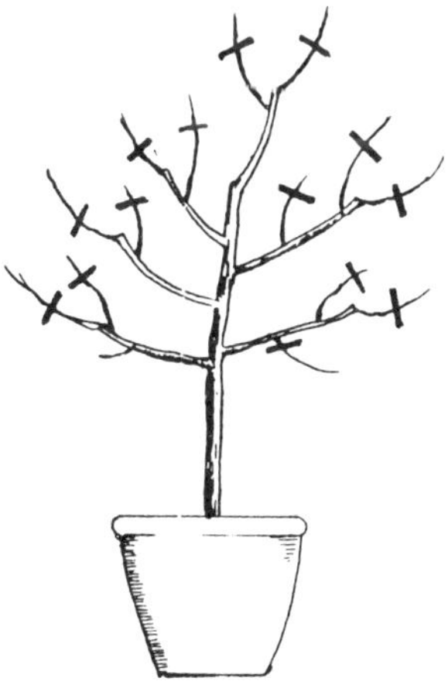

Training a compact leader tree for container grown fruit trees

Formative pruning

For the sake of stability and ease of maintenance, free-standing container-grown fruit trees are often best shaped in a roughly pyramidal form. Progressively shorter branches coming off a straight main trunk give the 'Christmas Tree' shape of the Compact Central Leader.

At planting, cut the central stem back to 1 metre if greater. Develop the bottom layer of the pyramid by retaining a pair of branches at a convenient height when the tree is in its pot—perhaps around 50 cm (1′ 8″) from the ground. (When purchasing, choose your tree carefully with this in mind.) Leave this pair uncut. Forcing them to grow horizontally, using spreaders or by pegging them down, will make them more fruitful. Remove all other branches growing above this lowest layer.

In the next and subsequent years, develop the next layer of the tree by selecting a further pair of branches some 50 cm (1′ 8″) above the last pair. Leave the newly selected pair uncut, but remove branches growing off the central trunk above them. Cut the lowest pair of branches back to around 30 cm (1′). Develop the tree in this manner each year until the required height is reached. Each layer of branches should be a little shorter than the one below.

Potted apple trees should be trained into this shape, but other fruit trees can also be trained this way or else shaped in a way that keeps them reachable and stable, retaining the type of wood that bears the fruit and allows sufficient light and air to penetrate. Some trees, for example the quince, medlar and the pomegranate, are both picturesque and fruitful when left unpruned and will give small, well-shaped but miniaturised trees when grown in containers.

Container-grown espaliered trees and those grown against walls should be trained as would trees in the ground. See Chapter 4 for instructions.

Companion Planting

Companion planting involves growing together plants that benefit one another, or at least where one benefits the other. This is often because one of the plants is disliked by some insect pest or disease that bothers the other. Sometimes, though, the benefit is due to some more mysterious, less easy to identify reason—possibly due to the mobilisation of some needed nutrients by each for the other, or perhaps to some shared microflora, or perhaps more pleasingly put down to 'liking one another's company'.

Companion planting seldom produces fast-acting effects and it may take several seasons before its full benefits are felt. It rates a mention here because it can reduce the amount of maintenance that a garden requires by reducing the need to spray for insect pests, or to treat the soil for disease-causing organisms. It may even reduce the amount of fertiliser needed for some crops. And, of course, it is a far more healthful approach to pest control, both for you and the environment.

Some of the more widely accepted 'Companion Plant' combinations are:

Chives, garlic, shallots and other members of the onion family (*Allium* species) are said to repel many insect pests, including aphids on roses. Chives help prevent apple scab and improve both the growth and the flavour of carrots. Onions improve the growth of beets, strawberries, tomatoes, lettuce and members of the cabbage family. All alliums inhibit the growth of peas and beans.

Marigolds (*Tagetes erecta*) help to control soil nematodes, which attack various crop plants and ornamentals.

Nasturtiums (*Tropaeolum majus*) keep down aphids when planted amongst broccoli and protect against woolly aphids when grown under apple trees. They enhance the growth of potatoes, cucumbers, radishes and members of the cabbage family.

Sage (*Salvia officinalis*) repels the white cabbage moth, that bane of the brassica family, and makes cabbages grow more succulent and flavoursome. It is a bad neighbour for cucumbers.

Lawn Plants—Grasses and Non-grasses

There are many different lawn plants available—but most of them are grasses. Commercial lawn seeds are usually mixtures of different types of grasses, sometimes with clover thrown in. Different grasses will grow best under different conditions and may look their best in different seasons. Winter grass, for example, flourishes in the cold weather, but dies off come summer; in contrast, couch grasses grow vigorously in the warm weather, but brown off in winter. Some grasses cope with shade, while others will tolerate drought. Buy cut turf or seed of a type/s that will suit your conditions and soil type. If you live anywhere near a large garden centre that offers a wide variety, it is worth travelling to be able to choose from a wide selection.

All of the grass lawns currently available for the home gardener will need frequent cutting; biological control is seldom an option and fortnightly mowing is usually necessary. A variety of couch that needs less frequent mowing is currently used in bowling greens, but is not available to the general public.

If you wish to have a non-grass greensward, your choice could be a herbal lawn of prostrate herbs such as Chamomile (*Anthemis nobilis*) or Creeping Thyme (*Thymus serphyllum*) for sunny spots, and Penny Royal (*Mentha pulegium*) for the shade. These will stand only light traffic, but give off their fragrance when walked on. There are a number of varieties of *Thymus serphyllum* available. Think twice before planting these herbs if you are allergic to bees, for their flowers will attract them; if opting for a chamomile lawn, be sure to obtain the non-flowering cultivar *Anthemis nobilis* 'Treneague'. The herbs are sold as tube stock. Mulch between plants while the lawn is establishing. Mowing will probably be necessary once or twice a year.

A Dichondra lawn will take a moderate amount of traffic, but is hard to establish. It is a temperate climate plant, and is available as seed from larger garden centres. The seeds should be sown into seed trays placed in the sun, then small clumps of the seedlings planted out when they are large enough to transplant. Dichondra (*Dichondra micrantha*) prefers a sandy soil, but even given ideal conditions, it may still curl up its toes and die. If it takes, it provides an excellent lawn, and will need mowing only occasionally, perhaps twice a year, depending on growing conditions. Once again, mulch between clumps at planting.

Lippia (*Phyla nodiflora*) is a drought-resistant grass 'substitute' that requires a warm climate; it, too, will take light traffic. It is available in clumps from larger nurseries in the hotter regions of the country. Again, mulch until the plants grow together to provide a cover for the soil. Lippia also bears bee-attractant flowers which can be removed by mowing.

Designing with Plants

I have refrained so far from offering advice on design beyond the functional, and I make no great departure from this now. It should be clear by now that I believe that people should have their gardens the way that *they* like them, rather than how someone else thinks they ought to be. For those who are still finding out just what it is that they like in a garden, or for those, like myself, who never tire of looking, there is a wealth of books available on garden design, ranging from the very practical to the purely inspirational. There are one or two situations often encountered by retirees, namely moving to a smaller space, and moving from a temperate climate to the tropics which even the most knowledgable gardener may have little experience of. I have some advice to offer for these situations.

Designing for a small garden

Dealing with a small space may require a radical re-think for those who are used to larger gardens. Most gardeners seek to make the space look bigger than it really is; the following tips should help to this end:

Firstly, keep everything in scale with the small space. Use plants with small leaves, small flowers, slender trunks and branches throughout the garden, including any functional plants such as hedging or creepers—for example, box, holly or a jasmine. Large features tend to draw the eye and cause the garden to shrink to just these eye catchers. This applies also to landscaping features. For example, large paving stones in a small garden emphasise the contrast and tend to dominate; use them only if they are to be a prominent feature. Smaller unit paving, such as paving bricks, will usually be a better choice.

Large trees are quite out of proportion—stick to smaller growing species; there is no dearth of these. If your garden is sunny, choose from among the many varieties of flowering plums or cherries (*Prunus* species), crab-apples (*Malus* species), the smaller eucalypts with delicate leaves, or any of the small growing fruit trees listed above in the section on container-growing (although quince fruits may be a little large, if scale is all we are considering). If your garden is shady, choose from amongst the Japanese maples (*Acer palmatum*), the dogwoods (*Cornus* species), or the plants listed below.

Secondly, play tricks with perspective. Use the fact that things look smaller in the distance to your advantage: plant the furthest boundary of the garden with fine-textured plants (small-leaved plants with twiggy branches), while plants in the foreground can be on a larger scale. Colour can be used to emphasise this contrast as well: warm colours advance while cool colours recede, so restrict your most distant plants to quiet blue or purple-flowered specimens, or, best of all, just plain green. This, however, is complicated a little by the fact that strong contrasts, too, tend to 'come forward'. Thus a *bright* cool colour will not recede as it ought—just take a look at the purple flowers of the Lasiandra (*Tibouchina urvilleana*) to see this effect for yourself. Many of our natives are of fine texture and gentle hue and are useful in boundary plantings in this situation. Choose suitable plants for your site from amongst the wattles (*Acacia* species), honey myrtles (*Melaleuca* species), teatrees (*Leptospermum* species), grevilleas, and eucalypts or the lovely Geraldton Wax and its relatives (*Chamelaucium* species). Alternatively, grow either one of the exotics listed below. All will give a misty, indefinite, far away look to your boundaries.

Finally, take advantage of the vertical space within your garden. Disguise your boundaries with fine-textured climbers and trees that reach for the skies, and dress them down with progressively smaller plants until the area you have allocated to garden beds has been filled. This vertical layering directs the eye up and out and masks the limits of the garden.

Keep these three principles in mind, and you will be surprised at how filling your garden with plants can increase the sense of space.

Fine-leaved evergreen shrubs and trees for the small garden

There are many fine-textured evergreen trees and shrubs for this situation. Some have already been listed in previous sections, where attention has been drawn to their texture. Below are two other small trees. They are both light-growing and are at their most effective when used in combination with a fine-textured screening plant. Both are available as advanced plants.

Azara microphylla (Box-leafed Azara) Chile
8×5 metres (26′×16′) Temperate and subtropical
This small tree has weeping sprays of tiny little leaves and an elegant open habit. Tiny, inconspicuous flowers are produced in the winter and have a delicious and pervasive vanilla fragrance. Semi-shade; shade

Pittosporum 'James Stirling' Garden origin
5×3 metres (16′×10′) All regions
This cultivar of the New Zealand native *P. tenuifolium* has slender, almost black branches and tiny, silvery green leaves. Its delicate appearance belies its cast-iron constitution. A variegated form 'Stirling Mist', with cream markings on the leaves, gives an even softer appearance.
Sun; semi-shade

A 'temperate climate garden' in the tropics

Over the last decade or so in Australia, there has been a movement of retirees away from the cold southern States to the warmth of the tropical north. While few complain about the reliable warmth and the high annual rainfall of their new homes, some sorely miss the temperate climate gardens. While there are cold-climate plants that will not grow in warmer regions, in some cases there are equivalent plants that are native to the tropics and yet have the same 'feel' in hot areas as their temperate climate cousins. An example of this is the Vireya Rhododendron, from the near tropics in New Guinea, Indonesia and Malaysia. This 'feel' has to do with the size, colour and firmness of the foliage to a large extent.

Tropical plants are often large-leaved, with soft, fleshy, green foliage, and tend, like water in a vessel, to take the form of the space they find themselves in. Flowers too, are large, luxuriant and usually bright. All this is a result of the low-light, high competition situation that tropical rainforest plants have evolved in. Temperate climate plants, in contrast, generally have smaller firmer leaves and overall a more definite form. Leaves are more likely to come in shades other than green, while the flowers are smaller and often of gentler hue. However, there are exceptions to these rules, and the clever use of these exceptions can give the impression of a temperate climate garden in the hotter regions, or the impression of a tropical rainforest in the cold old south.

The constant heat of a tropical climate is often not a problem for temperate climate garden plants. Many originated in areas such as the Mediterranean region, Asia Minor, or the prairies of the United States and have evolved in a climate with very hot summers; they are well equipped to cope with the heat. It is, rather, the high rainfall that can prove their undoing in the tropics. They are adapted to the arid conditions that prevail in the summer in their country of origin, and simply cannot cope with constantly wet soils. While some may have persistent and unsightly disease problems due to the high humidity, increasing the drainage is the key to success with growing many of these plants in the moist heat of our northern regions.

There are a number of ways to achieve effective drainage. Firstly, the plants can be grown in containers using a free-draining growing medium. Individual pots can be used, or a self-contained raised garden bed can be built as discussed in Chapter 5. Or the garden bed can be built up less formally above the prevailing level so that the water runs off quickly, and the soil stabilised using rocks, groundcover planting or a mulching material that does not retain excessive moisture. A large quantity of gritty material added to the bed and/or large bore subsurface drainage can be installed in the garden to ensure prompt removal of excess water from the root zones of your plants.

Some southerly favourites such as roses, camellias and abutilons are riddled with problems in areas of high humidity and should only be attempted in the tropics where there is good air movement, such as in the highlands. There are 'temperate climate' plants that grow happily in the tropics, plants which, both by their appearance and their long association with cooler climes, impart a 'temperate' feel to any garden in which they are grown. Such plants include the butterfly bush (*Buddleia davidii*), the jacaranda (*Jacaranda mimosafolia*), the Mexican mock orange (*Choisya ternata*), the heliotrope (*Heliotropium peruvianum*), the nasturtium (*Tropaeolum majus*) and the petunia (*Petunia* × *hybrida*). Space does not permit a comprehensive listing of such plants here; the gardener will be better served, in any case, by books written specifically on gardening in the tropics. Many Australian plants, too, commonly found in southern gardens have tropical counterparts which resemble their more familiar temperate climate cousins. Such plants include the wattles, she-oaks, gums, paperbarks, bottle brushes, grevilleas and wonga-wonga vines, to name but a few. Australian plant enthusiasts will find no lack of familiar-seeming plants.

I hope this book has been of help in guiding your thoughts and actions towards a smooth passage to gardening into retirement. May your garden bring you joy, hope and wonder for many years to come.

Useful Addresses

Organisations

The Banksia Centre Gardens
The Therapeutic Horticulture Officer
Australian National Botanic Gardens
GPO Box 1777
Canberra
ACT 2601
Ph: (06) 250 9450 (from August 1997: (02) 6250 9450)

Horticultural Society of NSW
250 Blaxland Rd
Ryde
NSW 2112
Ph: (02) 9808 8392

Horticultural Therapy Association of Victoria
585 Waverley Rd
Glen Waverley
VIC 3150
Ph: (03) 9803 0133

Independent Living Centres, Australia-wide:
Canberra
ILC
Parkinson St
Weston
ACT 2611
Ph: (06) 205 1900 (from August 1997: (02) 6205 1900)
FAX: (06) 205 1906 (from August 1997: (02) 6205 1906)

New South Wales
ILC
600 Victoria Rd (PO Box 706)
Ryde
NSW 2112
Ph: (02) 9808 2477
FAX: (02) 9809 7132

Queensland
ILC
Newdegate Street
Greenslopes
QLD 4120
Ph: (07) 3394 7471
FAX: (07) 3394 1013

South Australia
ILC
180 Daws Rd
Daw Park
SA 5041
Ph: (08) 8276 3455
FAX: (08) 8276 7417

Tasmania
46 Canning Street
Launceston
Tasmania 7250
Ph: (03) 6334 5899
FAX: (03) 6334 0045

Victoria
ILC
52 Thistlethwaite St
South Melbourne
VIC 3205
Ph: (03) 9254 5400
FAX: (03) 9696 1956

Western Australia
ILC
3 Lemnos St
Shenton Park
WA 6008
Ph: (09) 382 2011 (from May 1997: (08) 9382 2011)
FAX: (09) 382 2896 (from May 1997: (08) 9382 2896)

Occupational Therapist—Horticulture:
Ms Lynne Baker
223 McKean St
Fitzroy North
VIC 3068
Ph: (03) 9481 4759

Technical Aid to the Disabled (TAD):
ACT
PO Box 14
Lyons
ACT 2606
Ph: (06) 258 4040 (from August 1997: (02) 6258 4040)
FAX: (06) 258 4039 (from August 1997: (02) 6258 4039)

New South Wales
PO Box 108
Ryde
NSW 2112
Ph: (02) 9808 2022
FAX: (02) 9809 7670

Northern Territory
PO Box 41302
Casuarina
NT 0811
Ph: (08) 8945 4115
FAX: (08) 8945 3163

Queensland
PO Box 527
Annerly
QLD 4103
Ph: (07) 3397 7055
FAX: (07) 3397 9020

South Australia
PO Box 112
Eastwood
SA 5063
Ph: (08) 8261 2922

Tasmania
Room 107
Douglas Parker Rehabilitation Centre
31 Tower Rd
Newtown
TAS 7008
Ph: (03) 6278 2758

Victoria
PO Box 88
South Melbourne
VIC 3205
Ph: (03) 9254 5625
FAX: (03) 9696 5190

Western Australia
Suite 5
Westrade Centre
Cnr Newcastle & Lord Sts
Perth
WA 6000
Ph: (09) 221 1406 (from May 1997: (08) 9221 1406)
FAX: (09) 221 3366 (from May 1997: (08) 9221 3366)

Stockists—Tools

Mainstream Retailers

Wolf Tools
These tools are sometimes stocked by hardware stores and nurseries. These retailers may not carry a full range, but should have a product catalogue and are usually happy to order items in for customers. Alternatively, the products can be obtained from the main suppliers:

New South Wales
Garden Specialities
Ph: (02) 9484 9109

Northern Territory
Barnyard Trading
Ph: (08) 8932 3997

Queensland
International Traders
Cordelia St
South Brisbane
QLD 4101
Ph: (07) 3844 2926

South Australia
Woodchuck
Ph: (08) 8277 6677

Paul Munn's Garden Centre
Ph: (08) 8298 6721

Tasmania
United Hardware
Ph: (03) 6278 1699

Victoria (Australian Head Office)
City & Rural Gardeners
675 Canterbury Rd
Surrey Hills
VIC 3127
Ph: (03) 9899 5684
FAX: (03) 9899 5687

Western Australia
Puraclene Products
Ph: (09) 444 6211 (from May 1997: (08) 9444 6211)

Rehabilitation Suppliers
Most operate a mail order service. Some will supply to pharmacies on request.

Australian Capital Territory
RELPAR—use NSW Office—(Garden Gripper, Pistol-grip Handle, Long-handled Weeder, Easi Kneeler)

Surgical Orthopedic Services (Kneel N Sit)
Units 4&5; 56 Townsville St
Fyshwick
ACT 2609
Ph: (06) 280 7244 (from August 1997: (02) 6280 7244)
FAX: (06) 239 1281 (from August 1997: (02) 6239 1281)

New South Wales
Able Rehabilitation Equipment (Kneel N Sit)
30 Prince William Dve
Seven Hills
NSW 2147
Ph: (02) 9674 1677
FAX: (02) 9674 6570

RELPAR: (Easi Kneeler, Baronet Weeder, Garden Gripper, Pistol-grip Handle)
48–52 Sydenham Road
Marrickville
NSW 2204
Ph: (02) 9519 2943

Queensland
Colletts Home Nursing Supplies (Peta Fist-grip Garden Hand Tools)
52 Price St
Nambour
QLD 4560
Ph: (074) 41 7588 (from October 1996: (07) 5441 7588)

L&M Equipment (Kneel N Sit)
260 Southpine Rd
Enoggera
QLD 4051
Ph: (07) 3355 4577

Màygar Medical (Pistol-grip Handle)
PO Box 23
Coopers Plains
QLD 4108
Ph: (07) 3344 2744

Morris Surgical (Long-handled Weeder, Garden Gripper)
124 Lutwyche Rd
Windsor
QLD 4030
Ph: (07) 3394 2000

Tasmania
RELPAR—Use Victorian Office (see below)

STATEMED Pty Ltd (Kneel N Sit)
18 Mertonvale Circuit (PO Box 126)
Kingston
TAS 7051
Ph: (002) 29 4733 (from November 1996 (03) 6229 4733)
FAX: (002) 29 3676 (from November 1996 (03) 6229 3676)

Victoria
RELPAR—(Kneel N Sit, Easi Kneeler, Baronet Weeder, Garden Gripper, Pistol-grip Handle)
17–19 Roberts Avenue
Mulgrave
VIC 3170
Ph: (03) 9546 1511

R. E. Ross Centre (Kneeling frame, especially asymmetrical model)
Caulfield General Hospital
294 Kooyong Rd
Caulfield
VIC 3162
Ph: (03) 9276 6234

Western Australia
KDB Engineering (Garden Grippers, Kneel N Sit, Pistol-grip Handle, Easi Kneeler)
1 Booth Place
Balcatta
WA 6021
Ph: (09) 344 2633 (from May 1997: (08) 9344 2633)
FAX: (09) 345 1237 (from May 1997: (08) 9345 1237)

Private Inventors/Small Manufacturers (Listed under product name)
Ascender Lift Barrows
3 Markham Lane
Ashfield
NSW 2131
Ph: (02) 9890 6690
FAX: (02) 9689 1300

Aussie Hoe
Ryan Household Products
Box 50
Warracknabeal
VIC 3393
Ph: (053) 98 2244 (from November 1997: (03) 5398 2244)

Ergonomic Shovel (Mail Order)
Peter Fegan
Botanic Niche Landscapes
PO Box 1314
Stafford
QLD 4053
Ph: (018) 889 039 or (07) 3350 2861
FAX: (07) 3852 1243

Garden Gillie
Victoria
Ph: (03) 9836 2682
FAX: (03) 9287 1602

New South Wales
Ph: (02) 9489 5466

HOSE HOLDERS:
1. Quick Step Products (Split ring hose holder)
   112 Gloucester Ave
   Belair
   SA 5052
2. G. B. Wallace & Associates (Forgecraft clamped hose holder)
   Suite 4
   158 Pacific Highway
   North Sydney
   NSW 2060
   Ph: (02) 9955 4316
   FAX: (02) 9955 0269

MET-A-LITE GARDEN STOOL:
Met-a-Lite Manufacturing Co Pty Ltd
17–19 Mitchell Rd
Brookvale
NSW 2100
Ph: (02) 9905 3947/2213

TANYANA EASY WEEDER:
Tanyana Pty Ltd
2 Marshall Ave
Pinjarra
WA 6208
Ph: (09) 531 1864 (from May 1997: (08) 9531 1864)
FAX: (09) 531 2179 (from May 1997: (08) 9531 2179)

UNIVERSAL BACK-SAVER:
Metroson
Tuggerah
NSW 2259
Ph: (043) 52 2614 (from August 1997: (02) 4352 2614)

Mulch

EZI-WOOL MULCH IN A ROLL (Mail order or pick up from Tom Garner)
Garner the Gardener
PO Box 50
Ringwood
VIC 3134
Ph: (03) 9876 2723

Select Bibliography

Baxter, Paul 1991, *Fruit for Australian gardens*, Pan Macmillan, Sydney.

Burnett, J. 1990, *Making your garden grow*, Lothian, Melbourne.

Clayton, Sandra 1994, *The reverse garbage mulch book*, Hyland House, Melbourne.

De Vaus, Peter 1988, *Vegetables for small gardens and containers in Australia and New Zealand*, Hyland House, Melbourne.

Elliot, W. Rodger 1984, *Pruning, a practical guide*, Lothian, Melbourne.

Green, Michael 1989, *Building for the garden*, Lothian, Melbourne.

Smith, K. 1990, *The backyard organic garden*, Lothian, Melbourne.

Index